THE RUNNER

Also by P.R. Black

The Family
The Beach House
The Long Dark Road

THE RUNNER

P.R. Black

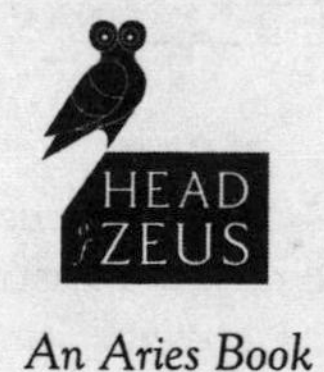

An Aries Book

This edition first published in the United Kingdom in 2021 by Aries,
an imprint of Head of Zeus Ltd

Copyright © P.R. Black, 2021

The moral right of P.R. Black to be identified as the author
of this work has been asserted in accordance with the Copyright,
Designs and Patents Act of 1988.

All rights reserved. No part of this publication may be reproduced,
stored in a retrieval system, or transmitted, in any form or by any
means, electronic, mechanical, photocopying, recording, or otherwise,
without the prior permission of both the copyright owner and the
above publisher of this book.

This is a work of fiction. All characters, organizations, and events
portrayed in this novel are either products of the author's imagination
or are used fictitiously.

A CIP catalogue record for this book is available
from the British Library.

9 7 5 3 1 2 4 6 8

ISBN (PB): 9781800246355
ISBN (E): 9781789543131

Cover design ©Lisa Brewster

Typeset by Siliconchips Services Ltd UK

Printed and bound in Great Britain by
CPI Group (UK) Ltd, Croydon CR0 4YY

Aries
c/o Head of Zeus
First Floor East
5–8 Hardwick Street
London EC1R 4RG

www.headofzeus.com

For Angie

1

Hey. You awake? All right in there?

Not too cold, are you?

Sorry it's taken so long. I won't keep you in suspense much longer.

Don't worry, I'll tell you where you are in a second.

Now, look… There's no need for that. I told you when we set off. Please don't… Look. I'll let you out, OK? Just don't kick the panelling. Did you know this van has been to Afghanistan? That's what the guy told me, when I bought it off him. Seemed to think this was a unique selling point. Hah! Please, show a bit of respect to the old girl, OK?

Calm down. I said calm… down. I will let you out. And I'll untie you. That's a promise. No joke, all right? It's not a trick. Definitely a trap, though. Heh heh.

Look… I don't have earplugs. Don't scream. Point one, it's not very nice. Point two, there is no one here to help you. Understand? No one's coming. There is no one here but you and me. Point three… you'll need to save your energy. It's really, really important. This is serious. Your life depends on it.

Ah. That's got your attention. Great! Now you're settled, I can tell you a bit more about where you are.

Listen. You hear that sweet sound? Isn't it grand? Takes me right back, I tell you. Funnily enough it makes me think of a painting my granny had in her bathroom. What does that sound suggest to you? Where do you reckon we are?

Hello? That was a question. It requires an answer. Would you like me to come in there and squeeze one out of you?

That's right – the seaside. Good. You're switched on. Back in the zone. Great. You need to be alert. You have to be focused. And you have to listen to what I'm saying to you. There are important points for you to pick up.

You are at the seaside. Lovely smell, too, eh? Maybe a little bit rank, at this stretch of coast, but never mind. Can't have everything. We're on a nice quiet stretch of the coast. There's an old pier maybe a mile and a half down the road, heading south... that's to the right, as far as you're concerned.

It's funny, I've driven past this way a few times. Someone's hanged old stuffed toys from the outside railing of the pier. Just let them dangle in the wind, there. If you didn't know they were there, you'd probably call the cops. From a distance a few of them look real!

Do you know how lucky you would need to be for someone to actually do that, right here, today? You'd be the luckiest girl in the world.

Anyway, the pier is your target. Got that? You're heading south, down the beach, to the right as you come out of the van, towards the pier. The tide's coming in, but you needn't worry about that.

Keep the pier in mind. Got it? It's an old, rickety pier. Part of it got burned. You used to get dossers bedding down for the night, but there's no one there now. The council sealed it all up. But there's a board loose in there. I need you to get into it. Or I should say... you need to get into it. You'll see the loose board when you get there. If you get there.

You with me? Taking this all in? I need an answer – yes or no.

What's that?

Good. You're listening. We're at the...? That's right. And you're heading to the...? Great! You know, you might be all right. You might do well out of this. You'll be right as rain.

Now. I'll open the door in a few moments. I can actually see what you're doing, right now. There's a webcam on you... No, don't bother looking for it. Take my word for it. So that stupid stance you're taking up, in front of the door, as if you're going to kick me when it opens... Not going to help. I'll finish you right there. So back up. That's it. Up on your haunches. Slide your knees up, under your chin... You're a very flexible lass, I must say. Bet you kick like a dray horse, as well! I chose you well, my love. I chose you very well.

As I said, I'm going to cut the cable ties, and you're going to be released. No trick, no joke. I'll have to use a knife to do it, so don't freak out.

Now, it's a dull day, not too sunny, but you've been in there in the dark for quite a while, so brace yourself, all right? Hang on... Three, two, one...

There we go!

Sorry. I did warn you.

Now, don't be getting upset. The mask is just for show, all right? I know, I should have warned you. Don't worry. Shut your eyes for a moment, take a few deep breaths. All about conserving energy, at this stage. Focus. You're into your fitness. You know how this goes. A runner, hey? You're a big strong lass. And you've got the gear on, hey? The right gear is so important, I find. Or equipment, in my case.

OK, here's the knife... I know, I know, this looks awful. But I promise, I'm only using this to cut the ties... Let's not be silly. Stop it now. Don't struggle.

I said don't struggle!

Sorry. I don't want this to be harder for you than it needs to be. OK? I'm cutting the ties. Once they're cut, don't move. You might think you can make a run for it, but I will be forced to do nasty things if you don't... That's good. Stay still. Great. Almost there... And done! Simple as that. I bet you're thinking, 'I wish I'd had my own knife, I'd have been out of here in a jiffy!'

OK, bad joke. Right. Here it is. You've got to run. That's the element I didn't take you through first of all. You have to run for it. Fast as you can. I will give you a twenty-second start. I'll let you get your circulation back. You can even warm up for a bit. There's a bottle of water on the floor, there. I won't completely hobble you.

Now, when I catch up with you, this is what I'm going to use. I'll use it to chop you up into tiny bitty pieces.

Crying won't help you. Nothing will help you. But you still have a chance. Got it? Focus. Be strong. Be fast. Part of me wants you to get away. You understand? I like winners. I want you to be a winner.

You get to the pier before I get to you, you're free. I'll run back to the van, and I'll be off. Then you can make your escape as you see fit.

You make for the sea, I'll get you. With this. See it? Don't look so shocked. Yes, it's real. And it's loaded. See?

You make for the rocks and the scrub, and try to get up the hill, or hide somewhere… ditto. I'll drop you. Be a dawdle for me. I'm good from any distance. Believe it.

Those are your choices. You're lucky to have choices, aren't you?

Some folk in your position get no choice, look at it that way. Let's be philosophical.

Look, I've drawn a line in the sand. Take your time to get warmed up… That's it! You get the idea. You have to be ready. Because there are no second chances. It's this or nothing. Got it?

Good.

Now get ready.

Now run. Run…

RRRRUNNNNNNNNNNNNNNNNNNAHHHH…

2

Deep breaths; in and out, in through the nose, out through the mouth. Prepare. Focus. Find the target.

Freya Bain stood still at the mouth of the alleyway, taking a breath, and preparing to run.

As alleyways went, it was somewhat genteel. It ran between two ranks of smart houses, built in the past twenty years or so, three- and four-bedroom units for families with toys and mobiles visible through the windows. It was a genuine pathway to the canal, and the park, and Freya's preferred running route – it wasn't a place of skips, bins, and even more unspeakable refuse, the places from the city centre threaded through with grim invertebrate piping undulating along the brickwork, the guts of the buildings strewn around the back where no one could see it. This was a smarter place, bordered with largely unvandalised fencing, a place where you hardly ever saw anyone. But it was still an alleyway, and still lonely.

She fed the earbuds into her tiny ears, cued the playlist, stretched her troublesome calf muscle one more time, and began the run.

Even if the sun was high in the sky, this opening section was dark and foreboding. A willow tree fifty yards down had even been cut back earlier in the spring, but it had now come into leaf. Freya had to angle her shoulders and let it pass, one single frond tickling her cheek. Someone could have been hiding there, and her imagination actually placed someone in among the tree, every time she passed. She wondered what her fitness tracker showed, every time she passed this place – a spike in the heart rate, until she was through.

Once through the ginnel and back out into the open, things got better; she had loosened off completely, and fell into a nice, steady rhythm. There was only the odd dog walker around here, as the houses backed onto a play area, one of those combination football pitch/basketball places, which did not have people playing either. One Friday evening there had been drunken teens. Freya had shied away from getting her trainers on after that, on a Friday.

The play area gave way to another slightly curved path, and then she was on the canal bank towpath at last. This was dodgier terrain, with many things to avoid in her path. The dog waste bags were somehow most offensive of all – at least mother nature could deal with the shit, she reasoned, but not the bags – and there was sometimes broken glass to contend with, or large puddles sunk into the rough, pitted surface, kneaded and bubbled like modelling clay by the elements. Other runners and cyclists were common. She shared a nod with these as they passed – dressed in Lycra and neoprene like her, with trainers that could have been doing with an upgrade long before – although she did not recognise any of them. She knew the canal was a different prospect after dark, particularly when it skirted some of the rougher estates, but she didn't concern herself with those times. Late afternoon, when lunch had properly settled in her stomach, was best.

Before long she was into the zone. Freya disliked to hear about people talking about The Zone as some gym bunny's motivational phrase. In her mind, the zone was a place of sublimity, where she couldn't feel pain and she wasn't out of breath; when the impact on her joints and gravity's remorseless tug were minor considerations. Today was one of the good days, one of the days where running became a habit, something to be enjoyed, not endured. Ducks scattered as she approached, taking to the water. A spindly black silhouette followed her through the turbulence as she pressed on.

Three K, four K, four and a half… she was barely out of breath, fully engaged in the tunes, but all too soon came the turn-off, back through another, scrubbier estate where young children out on their bikes had once spat on her as she passed. Once she was through here, she was back on the high street, past the shop where her mother used to send her for bits 'n' pieces, the businesses such as the Carpet Hatch and the fireplace outlet, which somehow still clung on to existence beside the vape shops and the internet café, which had devolved back into a simple café with the advent of smartphones. And finally, past the pub, which her mother had once owned, and the flat on top where she had once lived.

Freya put her head down and didn't look inside. It was the best way of guaranteeing no more pain, although it had only been two weeks. Two weeks since the hospice, and her mother turning that shade of yellow – Saturday morning cartoon yellow, unloved pepper at the back of the fridge yellow, the yellow of a boiled sweet that would suck out your fillings, something that couldn't be good for you. The promise that everything would be all right, when Freya knew it wouldn't.

She ran aggressively at the end, keeping up the endorphins. Fight the sadness, she thought. Fight the sickness. Hold it all back.

Freya was wheezing by the time she reached the new block of flats, the place where just about every window had been filled with a man leering at her as she directed the removals men – a smart enough place, but not populated by smart enough people. She slowed down to a jog before she turned into the cul-de-sac, fringed with black waist-high railings that cast the coat of a tiger onto the front of the building at night.

And it was here, with the security door in sight, as she had just stopped the playlist on her phone, with the sweat beginning to drop down her forehead and along the length of her nose, that the man jumped out at her.

'What the fuck?' she cried.

'Oh, sorry.' It was the postman – a bald man in his early forties who vaped constantly, every time Freya saw him pass the front of the building. Though it wasn't particularly warm he was wearing shorts and a pale blue short-sleeved shirt, with the mailbag looped over his shoulder. He looked genuinely chastened, holding out a hand. 'It's Ms Bain, isn't it? Flat 2/1?'

'Yeah... Sorry.' She smiled. 'I didn't mean to swear at you.'

'Don't you worry – I've been called worse on this job. It's my fault – shouldn't have startled you. There's a letter for you – you have to sign for it.'

Dismay clutched at her guts as he held out the Recorded Delivery letter. She recognised the letterhead, even upside down, as she signed the postie's keypad. It was from the solicitor. Today would be the day she would find out. Her mother's promise.

3

On Freya's mantelpiece, she kept one picture of her mother from healthier days – when Freya had been perhaps fifteen or sixteen. Mary Bain had been red-headed, and what they called 'big-boned', without meaning 'fat' – an Irishwoman with good strong cheekbones, fleshy where lots of men had liked it, and with quick, bright, blue eyes that could radiate mockery or mischief across an entire room. It was a contrast to the way she'd been near the end; it was the way Freya liked to remember her. There was a wicked twinkle in those eyes. It was the side of her mother she had loved best.

Freya took a deep breath and opened the envelope. It was from the solicitors. Her mother's will.

'We regret that you could not be present for the reading of the will. There follows a letter from your mother, enumerating her estate.'

The second section began, marking out her mother's will.

'Owing to policies put in place, I hereby leave all my belongings to my daughter, Freya, my only living relative. This includes an annuity of £5,000 pounds per year, guaranteed for ten years, as well as a lump sum of £22,000. On top of that, my daughter may not be aware that I actually purchased the family home, and the mortgage has been fully paid. I bequeath this flat to my daughter, as well as all my possessions therein.

'There is also £11,000 in Premium Bonds, which will automatically pass to her upon my death. There is also savings totalling £152,678, and the flat above the pub, which I leave to my daughter.'

Freya stifled a gasp, heart thudding. She had to wipe away some tears, pacing the room, before she could continue.

'Now comes the part that pertains to personal matters, and the answer to a question you have long asked.

'You have always asked me who your father was. I am sorry that I was never able to tell you. Being an orphan myself and raised by psychopathic nuns, I was painfully aware of the effects that a fractured family line can bring to a person. I know it can be alienating. I lied to you, and I feel a sense of shame. I told you your father was up in heaven. Later, as you grew older and more curious about the details, and then suspicious of my evasiveness on the subject, I told you a half-truth; that he was just someone I had known briefly.

'You took this to mean that you were the product of a one-night stand, and I was always proud of how well you dealt with this idea. Nothing fazed you at school, though I knew some people could be cruel. I always felt dreadful that you were an only child, that you never formed strong bonds with friends, that I couldn't even give you aunts and uncles and grandparents. It was always just you and me.

'But the truth is that your father is still alive. I know who he is, and where he is. I never told you when you were old enough to know, for a very good reason. Now I feel you should be told the truth. At the age of twenty-five, you deserve to know.'

Freya smirked. 'Typical,' she said aloud. 'Milking the drama all the way.'

'Your father is a man called Gareth Solomon. He is currently held in a category-A prison for murder, and there is no chance of him being released any time soon.'

The world began to constrict around her. Her heartbeat had surely never been so loud, bone-deep percussion in her ears.

'This name may not be a familiar name to you. He is more commonly known as the Woodcutter. I will spare you the details of what he was convicted of, but you will find a lot of this online. You may not want to read it all. Certainly, I took the shame of him and his deeds to my grave.'

Now Freya felt the horror. Freya had felt nervous about her father's identity before, but there was also excitement. Mary had told her that she would answer her 'question', and when it came to Freya and her mother, there was only one question outstanding. This had been exciting. Even if there was some scandal attached to the question of her paternity, or a secret that might have wrecked a happy family somewhere down the line, at least she would have known, at last, who her father was. But the picture had become horribly dark in a matter of seconds. The excitement had given way to dread. You didn't get a nickname like that for no good reason. Even if it was a moniker given to a sportsman for things he did on the field of play, it didn't augur well.

'He was a killer? My father is a fucking murderer?'

Hands shaking, she took up the letter again.

'I can't say that your father and I were in love. He was a regular at the pub I worked at before I went to the Tap. I did know him. He was handsome and I was lonely. It's one of those things that can happen. He was strange, but I won't admit to feeling anything negative about him. I did not divine that he was evil – I had no second sight or clairvoyance to call on. You're twenty-five, Freya, so you'll remember when you were twenty-one. I was young and I made a mistake. I wanted a child, though – you must understand that. You were wanted, you were loved, and that was and always will be true. He did not know about my pregnancy, because he moved on before I started to show. I heard news of his arrest when you were eight months old.

'Now you know the truth, you have to decide what you want to do with it. I kept this news from you and I did consider keeping it a secret. But then I wondered what might happen if you became curious. All the breakthroughs we have these days with DNA profiling and gene mapping, as well as family tree tracing might have given you an opening to find out about your father. Imagine how you would have felt, not knowing the circumstances, and knowing the Woodcutter was your father? But all the same, it was knowledge I wanted to hide from you, while I was alive. I hope you can understand; whether you do or not, I hope you can forgive me. I am truly sorry. But you are my daughter. He had no hand in your upbringing. I made no contact with him. It is unlikely he knows you exist. It is my hope that you never encounter him, given the crimes he committed. But you should know that he did not trick me, and that I did like him and I made the choice to be with him, long ago.

'My love to you, now and forever. Mary.'

Freya took up her phone, immediately. Who was he? The Woodcutter? She knew that name, somehow. A quick search on her phone brought the answer.

Images appeared in Freya's phone. Nineties hairstyles. Nineties make-up; bright red lipstick slashed across smiling faces. Not just women; a man was in there, too. All young. Trapped in analogue photography, coarse grain, faded colours. One or two school photos, a permanent fixture on a grandparent's mantelpiece. Unchanging but no longer an embarrassment.

Then the headlines. All of the same disturbing, dissonant tone. WOODCUTTER... MANIAC... CAGED... HOW MANY?

And his face, of course. A mugshot. No downwards-tilted chin, no sardonic expression, nothing like Alex from *A Clockwork Orange*. Just a frank, direct stare. Unabashed. Right into Freya's eyes.

And they were her eyes. Deep and black, not like Mary's. They caught the light in an unnaturally bright circle.

'God... I'll have to think... God...'

Then she actually did faint. It wasn't like a light being switched off, or a cartoon sock on the jaw. The world tilted; she might have forgotten to breathe.

4

The visit took a while to set up. First of all, there was the funeral to get through.

Freya thought there was a decent turn-out, mainly faces from the pub, some of whom Freya recognised. The priest made a fantastic job of pretending to know Mary, or care. He read out Freya's edited highlights of her mother's life as if he knew what he was talking about. She guessed that these guys had plenty of practice at this.

What touched Freya the most – finally dislodging the tears, and then the loud, embarrassing sobs, soaked up into the bosom of a worn old barfly who tried to smother her afterwards – was the practised dignity of the pall-bearers.

Among her mother's papers was Freya's birth certificate, and there, in the box outlining who her father was, confirmation of sorts. At least, confirmation enough to be able to approach the authorities without seeming like a crank.

Freya was told to put her request in writing when she emailed, then called the prison authorities; two of these missives, printed off at the local library, went unanswered. The third one was answered by the governor, who professed scepticism. Freya grew impatient, and repeated all that she knew.

'I have been told that your prisoner, Gareth Solomon, is my father. My mother's name was Mary Bain. She had a brief relationship with him. She wanted to keep his identity from me. Can you at least speak to him and let him know I want to make contact?'

Somebody, somewhere must have made the connection. After a fresh delay, the arrangement was made. First there was an interview with the governor of the prison, a surprisingly dainty little woman who put Freya in mind of a bird of prey – intense, focused, but easily startled. She made Freya uncomfortable; it was clear to the younger woman why and how she had become a governor.

'You understand what this man has done?' she said, never once breaking eye contact with Freya. 'You understand why he is locked up in here?'

'I've studied the cases,' Freya said.

'What – online? Wikipedia and such?'

'Sure. It's very detailed.'

'You still don't know the half of it.'

'I'm aware of what he's done.'

'And he is definitely the man named on the birth certificate?'

'You'll have to check with him, won't you?'

'He's said very little on the matter. I believe that's at the instruction of his lawyer.'

Freya took a breath. 'Well… there it is, in black and white. My mother swears it's him.'

'That hardly constitutes absolute proof, Freya.'

'Fine. Let's be sure about it – I can have it proven, or disproven, with a DNA test.'

'I can tell you that Gareth Solomon won't agree to it.'

'Then look into my eyes,' Freya said. 'Closer than you already have. Look deep into them. You see his eyes, don't you? You must see the resemblance. I take it you've met him in person?'

The governor angled her head, and ground her teeth. 'There is a strong resemblance. But that in itself…'

'Mention my name to him. Mention my mother's name – Mary Bain. It's all in the letter. There's every chance he'll remember. Even if he doesn't tell you as much. I want to meet him.'

The governor folded her hands, and sat up straight. 'Silly question corner. Why do you want to do this?'

'Silly answer – he's my father. I've a right to know who he is. I've a right to speak to him. I deserve contact. I've grown up with this mystery hanging over me. I… hated my mother for it, for a long time. I thought she was playing games. I used to wonder – was it one of the men in the pub? Was it someone she had loved? Was it a one-night stand? Now I know she was just protecting me.' Freya's voice broke. The governor offered her a tissue.

'I am truly sorry, Freya,' she said, in a kinder tone.

'I think it's time I made contact,' Freya said, finally. 'Wouldn't you do the same?'

'He's a multiple murderer.'

'That's never been proven, actually. He's been convicted of one murder. You've never been able to prove the rest. There isn't enough evidence. There aren't even any bodies.'

The governor steepled her fingers. 'He's been sentenced

for one murder, that's true. But the judge took into account the probability that he committed more. That's why he'll never be let out. There's not a Home Secretary born who would consider that. Do you know what he did, Freya? Really? He took girls – and a boy, too – roughly the same age as you, and…'

'As I said,' Freya said, growing irritated, 'I've done my research. Are you going to let me see my father? Or at least ask him if he'll agree to talk to me?'

The governor sighed. Freya never did find out her name. Apparently, it was the convention to keep it a secret, lest she should be targeted in some way on the outside. 'I'll look into it,' the woman said.

And she was as good as her word. After a number of delays, the event was set up. Freya arrived outside the prison in a taxi. It was one of those functional but intimidating Victorian buildings, complete with turret corners. It was an intricate, but forbidding building, like black teeth gnashing together. If Freya had been asked to draw a Category-A prison as a child, then it might have looked something like this building, complete with its high, jagged fence and searchlights. Inside, though, it was bright and modern. She had half been expecting catcalls and a sudden storm of flung piss, filtered through wire mesh strung tight overhead, but there was no sign of any inmates at the front desk, not any battery-hen-style cages for some of the country's most dangerous men.

They were expecting her; the governor came through, in a smart outfit that looked like velvet from a distance, and stark white earrings that resembled adhesive hooks for a cloakroom.

They were accompanied by two enormous men as they proceeded through a set of gates, once Freya had filled in the paperwork and her ID lanyard was hung about her neck.

'A word about your father,' the governor said, walking a step or two in front of Freya, and not looking back as she spoke. 'This isn't exactly going to be like *The Silence of the Lambs*. He won't be in a cage. He will be behind glass, but you'll be able to speak to him freely. An officer will be present. It should go without saying that you won't be able to pass anything to him, and if he says anything that we decide is untoward, then the interview will be terminated and you'll be asked to leave – no ifs or buts.'

'Fair enough.'

'That's the practical, hands-on stuff. Now a word about his conduct. How much do you know about the Woodcutter cases?'

'I've looked through most of them. I read Mick Harvie's book, too.'

'Mick Harvie.' The governor's delivery of these words was comical, as if uttering the name of a mortal enemy.

'You've met him?'

'Unfortunately. Mick Harvie wrote a very sensationalist piece of work, Miss Bain. I wouldn't rely on his reporting as fact.'

'He does seem convinced that there were up to a dozen victims of the Woodcutter.'

'I would say that's on the extreme side, when it comes to how many he's suspected of killing.'

'How many would you say, then?'

The governor blinked before answering. 'I think your father killed six people, for certain. One or two others, we're not sure about. A few possibilities, but there's just not enough evidence to link him to those disappearances. Once a body turns up, we'll know.'

'But he was only convicted of one murder. And that was on circumstantial grounds, wasn't it?'

The governor stopped, as they approached a huge, no-messing steel door with a vast iron wheel in the middle. 'Have you been speaking to your father's lawyer? Cheryl Levison?'

'No. Never heard of her. What's his lawyer got to do with it?'

'Your father is consistently trying to engineer appeals against his conviction. Including one going through the system as we speak.'

'As is his right, surely?'

'Of course.' The governor sighed. 'Listen, Miss Bain. You're going to speak to a very unusual person. Whatever you've heard about him, or whatever you might think of him based on your interview, let me give you some advice: take everything he says with a whole truckload of salt. Gareth Solomon is a liar. It's part of his make-up; maybe circumstances made him that way. Maybe it's an ability he was born with. Maybe it's a talent he has that he's gotten down to a fine art. Nobody knows. But one thing I can tell you is that he's one of the most manipulative, persuasive people you'll ever meet. You might have read some stories in the press about his fan mail. You're not the only female visitor he's had. To say nothing of the letters we receive, on a weekly basis. He has the gift of the gab, you might say. So be warned – you should be on your guard, and you should tell him very little about yourself.'

'He's not a threat to me. Is he?'

'He might not be a threat, exactly, but he will seize on any detail and try to control you. That's part of his make-up. He's a manipulator, as well as a killer. You should imagine a Venn diagram of psychopathy and sociopathy. Gareth Solomon is in the area that overlaps with both.'

'I'll handle him.'

'You don't sound very sure of yourself.' Here, the governor smiled at last. 'Can I ask what age you are?'

'I told you – twenty-five.'

'I would have thought you were younger. You're old enough to be wise at twenty-five, that's for sure. Let's see how wise you can be, when faced with a man like Gareth Solomon.'

Freya smiled. 'Now, would *you* be trying to manipulate me, here, governor?'

'For your own good.' The prim little woman nodded to the guard, who opened the doorway. It swung open – slowly – onto a long, strip-lit corridor. A guard stood on the other side. He was standing to attention like a soldier with a bulging-eyed focus and determination.

The governor went on: 'Welcome to A wing. There are three serial killers housed here in total, including your father. They're all household names, you might say. I've heard that there is a bit of competition between them all, to see who's the most deranged. Your father is the winner, by all accounts.'

Perhaps it was having other killers mentioned in the same breath as him that finally soured Freya's adrenaline; now, in the narrowing corridor, there was dread. The figure she was about to meet was a shadow, even though she knew his face well by now. He might as well have appeared at the head of the corridor, and ran at them.

A voice that might have been her mother's said: *Just stop. Stop this. You don't have to do it. You don't have to know any more. Leave him to rot.*

But that's not good enough. I have to know. I've spent my whole life not knowing. And I've come this far. You didn't raise a coward, did you?

She took a deep breath, and quickened her pace.

Freya followed the governor up the corridor. There were no cell doors, here – she saw one room that seemed to have a squash court in it, empty except for a ball in the centre of the floor. Two prison officers sat at a canteen, bursting into sudden laughter at a comment one of them made; and finally, they came to another set of double doors, with an immense wheel in the door and yet another bulky prison officer.

'You'll be the only two people in the room, other than the guards. Please bear in mind all that I said, Miss Bain. Let him know nothing about you. And good luck.'

They shared an awkward handshake, before the governor nodded to the prison officer on the door. He was young and meaty with a crop of acne coming into flower on his chin, with blond eyelashes that cried out for eyeliner. But he was tall and strong, seemingly twice the size of Freya.

'Follow me, miss,' he said.

They entered into a tranquil room that reminded Freya of the oratory at her sixth form college, a place of sunlight filtered through long, thin drapes, with pine furniture and an oatmeal carpet. The end of the room was dominated by a long, thick plexiglass partition stretching all the way from the ceiling down to a desk, with black speaker units attached. On the other side of this plexiglass was another prison officer.

'I'll be sitting beside you,' said her own escort. 'I'll be quite close, so that can be off-putting. But it's for your own safety.'

'I understand.'

'Please sit down.'

Once Freya did as she was told, the prison officers shared a nod.

A door on the other side opened, and then Freya was face to face with her father, for the first time.

5

Freya had expected him to be taller. She had towered over her mother since taking a stretch in early adolescence, and had always assumed this quality had come from her father's side. However, he was bang average; five nine, no more.

She had expected an orange jumpsuit, too – perhaps even black and white stripes, or arrows up and down the arms – but he was dressed in a pair of jeans, a blue pullover with a blue shirt collar creeping out above the neckline. In terms of prison movie clichés, what he did have was a huge, muscular build, of the kind that Freya usually associated with juicers working on the doors or preening themselves by the free weights in the gym.

His head was shaven, which did not suit him at all, but he had a thick, black but well-kempt beard, which did. He might have been an old-time wrestler – British, not American, the stuff of celebrity appearances on ancient Sunday matinees and mean-spirited nostalgia TV retrospectives. Freya could picture old ladies sat in the front row, roaring at him.

Those eyes were unmistakable, though – liquorice-black pupils, almond-shaped eyes above a thin, slashed brow.

These eyelids contracted as he sat down, and gazed at her with cool intensity, his hands folded on the tabletop.

Freya folded her own arms in response, to hide the fact her hands were shaking.

He spoke suddenly, and she flinched. His voice was somewhat muffled by the effect of the microphone, but it was smooth, with a hint of languor. He might have been a sardonic, embittered schoolteacher smacking his lips over some stupidity among his charges. 'I have to say, if you're a fake, you're a good one.'

'I'm not a fake.'

'You look incredibly like my older sister. Which is to say, you look incredibly like me, and my dear dead mummy.'

'Of course I look like you. I'm your daughter.'

'So you say. You going to introduce yourself?'

'I'm Freya. You going to shake hands?'

He studied her for a moment through the glass, balefully, then snorted laughter. 'All right, that's a point to you. Good stuff. We might make some progress, here.' He leaned forward, and without blinking, placed a hand on his own chest. 'Gareth. Pleased to meet you. Now that we've got that out of the way… what can I do for you?'

'Do for me?' Freya was stumped. 'I don't want you to do anything.'

'I mean if you're looking for money, or…'

'I'm not looking for money,' she said, sharply.

'Or a place to stay…' He grinned, and gestured around about him. 'I'm all out of spare rooms.'

'I told you, I'm not looking for anything.'

'Then I'm afraid I don't understand. Why are you here?'

'Because… I'm your daughter.'

He sniffed. 'And…?'

'And nothing. That's why I'm here. I only found out in the last few weeks, after my mother died. She told me you were the father. You're named on the birth certificate. I wanted to make contact with you. I've a right to speak to my own father.'

'Yeah, and this intrigues me. I've never heard of you before. What did you say your mother's name was?'

'Mary Bain. She worked at the Jetty pub, in Rimesdale. You were passing through, but you ended up living with her for a few months. You had a relationship; you left when she became pregnant. It's possible you didn't know.'

'Mary Bain… it does ring a bell. And Rimesdale? I stayed in Rimesdale for a fortnight, I think, maybe three weeks…'

Anger flooded Freya. 'It's you. Don't waste time denying it. You and Mary were together. I'm your daughter. I'm giving you basic facts.'

Solomon had continued to speak over her, a finger placed on the dark hair mossing his chin. '…So many women, you understand. I mean you're an adult, right? Full-grown? I didn't always look like an extra in a grindhouse biker movie, I was a good-looking guy. You've seen the mugshot, haven't you?'

'Yes, I've seen the mugshot. It's not hard to find. As you've just admitted yourself, we're a close match.'

'You've made it hard to tell, in a lot of ways. With the eye make-up. Very striking. You know who you remind me of? Siouxsie Sioux. You know her?'

'No. I'm a full-grown adult, but I'm not geriatric.' She paused a moment, enjoying his bemusement. 'That was a joke. Of course I know who Siouxsie Sioux is. Thanks for the compliment. I think.'

'Ah, a comedian! A girl after my own heart. In a manner of speaking.' Solomon drummed his fingers on the tabletop. She couldn't remember him blinking or looking away from her once. 'It is a great big thumping coincidence in terms of times and dates, I must admit. And you do share a few of my features, my little cherub. Good strong jaw. The eyes, of course. Minus the mascara. Fancy that? I'm a father. Call me "daddy". This is a happy day for me, isn't it?' He angled his head towards the prison guard stationed over his shoulder, but the man remained totally impassive. 'You guys should break out the bubbly!'

Freya wanted to leave. As fishing trips went, this was a strange endeavour from the start. She had been primed for hostility, or outright denial. Instead, she felt she was being treated to a performance. She had no desire to play a bit part.

'So,' he continued, 'mummy dearest died, did she? Of what?'

'Cancer.'

'I'm sorry. Terrible way to go.'

'Not as terrible as some.'

'Quite quick, was it?'

'Reasonably. I can't decide if it was a blessing or a curse.'

'A blessing,' he said, all the levity disappearing. 'I've seen a couple of the guys in here get it. Smokers, you know. Idiots. You smoke, you know what's coming. But they can't stop. And don't want to. They just shrivelled up and died. Took eighteen months, in one case. One guy had throat cancer. Big tough guy, shoulders like a bison. He looked like something you'd crowbar out of a sarcophagus, by the time they let him out on compassionate grounds. If you get spared that, then it's something, believe me.'

'How do you feel about it?'

'About what?'

'About Mary Bain dying. You were together a little while. I presume you liked each other.'

Gareth Solomon sighed. 'This was all so long ago… I don't say this to hurt you or to get a reaction from you, but I struggle to recall. I moved around a lot at that time. Driving jobs here. Labouring there. Casual work in pubs – that's how I met her, I guess. I was a bit of a rover, and you can take that pejoratively if you like.'

'You don't remember her? Like… nothing?'

He raised a hand, sensing her growing distress. 'I think I remember her. Quite short? Blue eyes? Blonde? Or, she would have been blonde, at the time. Very good-looking. Cute – like a little dynamo? Long blonde bob, at one stage?'

'That's right. She preferred being a redhead, though. Colour changed now and again. But she had that style all her days, the bob. Right up to the end.'

'Yes, I remember her. She was…' He struggled for the word. When it slipped out, it felt grudged. '*Lovely*. She was just… lovely. It was a great time. The Nineties, eh? Doesn't the time fly? The mid-Nineties already feels like it was a million years ago. Summer of Britpop, that one. Very warm out, July or August. Pulp and Blur and Oasis. The Spice Girls a half-formed thought in some executive's head. Still to happen. Still to explode. Who were those boys – Supergrass? They were lots of fun. They'll be in their forties. They could be grandads by now. Great times. Is it me or is music rubbish nowadays? I don't get to hear much of it, but what I do hear… aw.'

'I don't mind Britpop. Not as good as some people say. Lot of landfill.'

'Landfill! I like that one.'

'Quite egalitarian, in a way… lots of girls in bands.' Freya was babbling, trying to make sense of what she'd been told, how the missing pieces fit in her own self-image. 'Did she ever visit you? Mary?'

'Not once. Absolutely not. Never wrote to me, either.'

'Do people write to you?'

'Sure. I'm not stuck for female contact, I'll say that much. Colin Lucas Stewart is one of my china plates in here. You might know him as the South Side Strangler. He wasn't a bad-looking guy, as it goes. But he is so bloody jealous over the sheer number of letters I get. You wouldn't believe it. I should hire a secretary. Married women, aunts, grannies, girlfriends. The things they *say*.'

The idea repelled her. Freya had come into this in a very natural state of curiosity, but not naivety. She wondered if younger people than her had tried to get in touch with the Woodcutter. 'Do you write back?'

'Well… I can't talk about my case, really. I've no idea who I'm talking to. Could be a copper or someone like that. Or even a relative of some of those poor people.'

'Poor people?'

'You know.' He shrugged. 'Victims.'

'*Your* victims?'

He smiled, and rubbed his chin again. 'Ah, let's not get into that. My lawyer says I'm not allowed to. Even if my long-lost daughter shows up.'

'This to do with your appeal?'

'Yep. All in hand. The law's changed. They'll let me out this time.'

'Yeah?'

'Oh, they will,' he said, without a pause. 'I know they will.'

'You seem very confident about that.'

'There's a reason for that, too.' He leaned forward. 'I'll break a rule. I'll go against what my lawyer said. Her name's Levison. Cheryl Levison. L-E-V-I-S-O-N. Get in touch, if you can.'

'What for?'

'Just listen carefully. Put the name in your phone. Or write it down, if you're old-school like me. You can find her on the internet. She'll fill you in.'

'About your appeal?'

'About the whole thing. And the reason why they'll let me out.'

'Any reason you can't talk about that now?'

'Not in any detail. But I can tell you the very simple reason that they'll have to let me out: I didn't do it. I'm not the Woodcutter. They've got the wrong man.'

'Time's up,' said the guard, at Solomon's side. He checked his watch, and the guard accompanying Freya mirrored the gesture.

'Gotta go. It's been fascinating. I guess you get to call me daddy.' Solomon grinned for the first time, showing even, if yellowed teeth. 'Remember: I didn't do it. I'm not the guy. And I will get out of here. We could meet up – spend some quality family time together.'

His facetiousness irritated her. As she got up to leave,

she said: 'Whatever happens, I'll be back. There's something that I have to know about you.'

He frowned. 'What's that?'

'The truth.'

And something changed in him, at that moment. His expression did not soften, exactly. It was as if his sardonic aspect had dropped, just for a second or two. Freya understood that his attitude and his manner were simply a defence, and possibly a flimsy one at that. He nodded at her, eagerly, and suddenly he looked unhappy. 'I'll tell you everything. In time.' He turned to the guard and nodded. The interview was over.

6

Back at the flat, Freya stared at the number at the top of her notepad.

She hesitated for longer than she would have liked to admit. Her hand poised over the phone, she remembered when she had first phoned a boy as a teenager; the feeling that her heart might have migrated to her ear, the sound waves of her pulse perhaps perfectly audible as the boy's father answered.

'Levison, Duke and Redman,' a woman on the end of the line said.

'Cheryl Levison, please,' Freya said.

'Can I ask who's calling?' After Freya gave her name, she heard the clicking of a computer keyboard. 'You're in luck. She's in. She's been expecting you. I'll patch you through. One moment.'

The holding music was far too loud. Freya held the handset away from her ear. Finally, an exasperated female voice cut it off. In the background there was social interference – loud voices, some of them raised in merriment. Was she in a pub?

'Ms Levison, I'm Freya Bain. I'm calling on behalf of my father.'

'You'll have to narrow it down, honey.'

She was abrupt, and Freya swallowed her diffidence and annoyance. 'I'm Freya Bain. My father is your client, Gareth Solomon. The Woodcutter.'

A brief, but significant pause. 'Wait there just a moment, would you? Don't go anywhere.' The holding music didn't return. Instead the background voices were muted, after a door was closed on them. Then came the sound of steady, assured footsteps, echoing up a long corridor. Freya imagined a dusty old courtroom, a space with cornicing and elaborate masonry that hadn't been cleaned for a while, staircases spiralling down to the cells below, or to hell. Then Levison spoke. 'The Woodcutter's daughter. Are you absolutely sure about that?'

'Certain of it. I'll happily prove it, if I can. He had an affair with my mother. She died a little while ago. She never told me who my father was. It's there, in her will.'

'I will need proof – what was it, Stella?'

'Freya.'

'Freya. Always liked that name. Always liked Stella, too. You know this is... Interesting. Very interesting. I'm preparing Gareth Solomon's appeal right now. This could be a very interesting thing. Well. Whether we can prove it or not, I'd be very pleased to meet you, Freya. You could be very helpful indeed.'

Freya knew not to trust her imagination. It had placed Cheryl Levison in a severe business suit, possibly still with her wig and gown on. Even so, she had expected someone severe, perhaps intimidatingly tall, like a female vicar but not one who would ever get invited on to do Thought For The Day.

Because of this, Freya walked past Cheryl Levison at first. They had been due to meet at a pub – a cocktail bar, in fact – which seemed quiet enough at lunchtime, but bore the signs and in some cases the scars of somewhere livelier once the sun went down. There was literally no one inside except for one girl behind the bar who never once looked up from her phone while Freya looked around. After a minute or two of confusion, Freya went back outside. Levison was there, at an outside table fenced off from the street. She was smoking, with a mobile phone held to her ear.

'Right back with you,' Cheryl Levison said into her phone. Then she hung up, and got to her feet, waving. 'Hey? Is it Freya?'

'That's right.'

'Come on up, honey.' She gestured to an entryway, usually roped off but left open in the afternoon sun. 'Don't be marching up and down the street all day on my account.'

She was intimidatingly tall – that part was correct. She also looked as if she was ready for a day out at the pub, in a black dress that seemed a little too short for the office. Freya wondered if she had been out all night, although the hair and make-up were too sharp for a dirty stop-out.

Thc lawyer was about fifty, and had looked after herself; she was blonde, with hair a little on the Nineties side, but it suited her. She was draped and garlanded with rings, brooches and chains that caught the light in painful slices, like morning sun on broken bottles. Good-looking, with warm dark eyes at odds with the harsh angles of her chin and cheekbones.

'Well, let's get a look at you,' Levison said, after shaking hands. 'Yep, I can see the resemblance, all right. Won't you sit down?'

'Thanks for agreeing to speak to me.'

'Not a problem. I can't stop long – got a meeting with a client just after two. I hope you haven't travelled far?'

'Train trip,' Freya said. 'Quiet, for a Wednesday.'

'Are you off work?'

'You could say that.'

'Ah. Compassionate leave.'

'No… Not really. I was made redundant, got a bit of money. I'm keeping my head down for a while. Checking out my options.'

'Oh. What's your line of work?'

'Phone farm, if I'm honest.' A giddy sense came over Freya; a chance to blurt out the truth. So she did. 'If I'm being double honest, I'm using this time to run. I'm a runner. Just for fun, not an athlete, or anything. It's an addiction, I guess. Something to help me get through the past little while.'

Levison had unlocked her phone already, and was texting while keeping up the flow of patter. 'I was so sorry to hear about your mother.'

Freya nodded.

'Now… exactly what is it you want?'

'Gareth said to contact you. Plus, I'm curious.'

That got her attention. Levison looked up from her phone. 'Go on.'

'About whether or not he did it. He says he didn't. And I can't be sure if he's lying or not.'

'Uh-huh. You'll forgive me if I ask you one or two questions, before we get into that. You say you're his daughter.

And – this was a little bit of a surprise – *he says* you're his daughter.' Levison peered at Freya. 'He seemed certain. I'm prepared to believe it. But I'd like to prove it, first.'

Freya shrugged. 'DNA is the key, isn't it? I can take a test. You got somewhere you want me to spit?'

Levison laughed, delighted. 'In fact, yep, I do – right here in this test tube. Better still, run the swab inside your cheek for me.' She fished out a sturdy vial from her handbag, unstoppered it, gently pulled out a swab, and handed it over.

Freya glanced at it, not sure if this whole scenario was a joke of some kind. Levison didn't even look away as Freya did as she was told. 'Excellent,' she said, resealing the test tube and sliding it back into her bag. 'You didn't hesitate. Well, not *too* much. That's a good sign.'

'There's no reason for me to hesitate. I'm his daughter.'

'How did you get on when you met him?'

'It was a little weird, as you'd expect. For him as much as me. It would have been weird in any case. Even if he wasn't in jail for murder.'

'He didn't commit murder,' Levison said, flatly. 'I can answer that question right now. He was fitted up for just one murder. There is no evidence to connect him with any others.'

'I understood there wasn't enough evidence to charge him. He was plenty connected to it, though.'

'Aren't you the smart kiddie?' Levison sipped at a coffee, coolly. 'So, why did you want to meet him?'

'Funny, he asked me the same thing. It's obvious, isn't it?'

Levison shook her head. 'Not immediately obvious, no.'

'Well… wouldn't you want to meet your father? If you suddenly found out who he was?'

'I suppose.'

Freya composed herself; every utterance from this woman left her wanting to respond with a cheeky remark. She heard an echo of her mother's irritation. *Too smart for your own good, madam. Learn to keep it buttoned.* 'He mentioned that he's quite confident about the appeal.'

'That's true. We may be preparing for a break in the case, in fact.'

'New evidence?'

'I can't say any more than that, of course. But we are trying to get your father out of prison. You could have a proper reunion.'

'I've done some reading on the case,' Freya said. 'The evidence against him seems watertight. He was seen in the area, getting into a car, near where the woman's body was found. Witnessed by one person. They seemed sure. That was the whole prosecution. Are you saying he didn't do it?'

Levison grinned. 'I don't think he killed June Caton-Bell. That's what he was convicted of.'

'What about the other disappearances? You don't think he's the Woodcutter?'

'As I said, I don't think he killed June Caton-Bell. Your father wasn't convicted of anything else, as I'm sure you know.'

'But they reckon one person is behind all five killings.'

'The fact is, the CPS didn't have enough evidence to charge your father with all five murders.'

'Doesn't mean he didn't do it.' Levison gave Freya a hard look, and didn't respond. 'Look, I'd just like to know. I don't know what to believe.'

'I wish I could tell you more. But one thing I can say is that your father didn't kill June Caton-Bell. Soon, we're going to be able to prove it. If he was convicted of the other four cases connected to the person known as the Woodcutter, then yeah – it would be harder to argue the toss. But as I should stress – your father was convicted of one count of murder only.' Levison frowned. 'Are you all right, love?'

Freya had faded out somewhat in a sudden chill. She pulled her coat tighter about her body. 'It's been weird,' she said, shivering. 'Just a lot to take in.'

Levison looked uncertain, for a moment. Finally, she reached out, and took Freya's hand in hers. 'I'm sorry, love.'

The street was quiet, even for a benevolent time of the day, after breakfast but well before lunch, and unseasonably cool. 'It's... Well... I lost my mother, and now...' She was going to say 'gained a father', but the wedding speech construction seemed ghastly, given the circumstances. 'There's so much I want to find out.'

'Bound to be odd.'

'Odd is my stock in trade.'

Levison slowly withdrew her hand, and took in Freya's clothes and dark hair. 'Just before we go... are there any other reasons you want to get in touch with my client? Any possible legal action?'

'I've already explained this. I wanted to make contact because I'm curious. No matter who he was, no matter what he's meant to have done. Wouldn't you be? Second... I have a doubt. I'm not sure he did it. I want to find out for sure.'

Levison didn't respond to that. Instead, she lit a cigarette. 'You want to go grab a drink?'

'No... Bit early.'

Levison angled her head. Her smile might have been painted on, her voice seething with irony. 'What are young people coming to? When I was… what age are you, honey?'

'Twenty-five.'

'Twenty-five… That's when you're old enough to call yourself an adult, with a straight face, I suppose. How boring. Anyway, when I was twenty-five, and a barrister offered me a drink or two, I'd have taken it.'

'I thought you said you were meeting a client?'

'That's right,' Levison said, brightly.

'No thanks. I'll grab a coffee later.'

The older woman shrugged, and took a long draw. 'Suit yourself. You know, you're *interesting*.' Levison's moist brown eyes focused on her for a second or two. 'Very interesting indeed. I like your style, incidentally. Love what you've done with your eyes. What is it you do outside of working in a phone farm, honey? You in a band?'

'No.'

'Sure? You look like someone famous. In a band. I bet you get that a lot.'

'Please don't say I look like Siouxsie Sioux.'

Levison frowned. 'Who the hell's that?'

'…Siouxsie and the Banshees?'

'Sorry, I think I peaked at Duran Duran. Never really kept in touch since. Full disclosure – I am still in love with Nick Rhodes. So, you're just… knocking around? Running, you said?'

'Just keeping myself to myself.' Which was true. And always had been. It never occurred to Freya that she was lonely; just alone. 'I was thinking of getting into journalism.'

'Journalism. Now that's a weird career. Especially the

parchment and quill wing. We all need it, we all read it, but that's a whole industry that's on death row. Fancies a dirty weekend in Dignitas. Don't tell me you want to be in newspapers?'

'Well, yeah,' Freya stuttered, more defensive than she'd anticipated. 'Like you say, it's an important job.'

'So much media's all done for us now, though. Clicks. The internet. Social media.'

'And that's why proper journalism's important.'

'Very true. So, you looking to study, you said?'

'I was. Part of me wants to make a more direct approach, though.'

Levison took a long draw of her cigarette. 'That's often the best way. And you don't have to study to be a journalist. I mean, there are things you have to know. *Sub judice*, that kind of thing. I'm assuming you can spell, and type really fast.'

There was something about this woman that got under the skin; she was being needled, but had no idea what purpose it served. 'As I say – I'm taking steps. I was lucky enough to inherit my mum's flat, and a little bit of money. So I'm assessing my options.'

'If you're breaking into journalism, then you might need a scoop. Something to break through with. You know what you can do? You can talk to a guy I know.' Levison fished out a battered moleskin-upholstered notebook, and riffled through to the back. She tore a sheet out, and handed it over. 'Here you are. There's a name to check. Give this guy a call.'

'Mick Harvie? Writer? What do you know about him?'

'Very famous man, in his field. What they used to call a crime correspondent. Like you, he's at a bit of a loose end.'

'I didn't say I was at a loose end.'

'That's true. You didn't have to.' Levison grinned. 'Give him a call. Say who you are. I think he'll be interested.'

Freya stuffed the torn sheet into a zip pocket in her jacket. 'Thanks. I think.'

'You're welcome.' Levison stubbed out her cigarette. 'Sure you won't have a drink? Last chance.'

'No thanks. I'd best be going. Thank you for your time.'

Levison got up, slipping the thin strap of her bag about her shoulder. 'I wouldn't bother with the coffee in here. Or the prosecco, come to think of it.' Levison winked as she put on a blazer. 'Must dash. I think we'll speak again, Freya. Sooner rather than later. I've got your number. I'll be in touch.'

7

Mick Harvie's house was at the end of a farmer's field left fallow. Sparse green spaces were overgrown with cornflowers with their heads turned away from Freya, while much of the churned earth surrounding these were seeded with stones. A dusty brown path, cracked in the warm sunshine, led all the way to a place that was called 'The Pines', for no good reason. Had there been pines anywhere near that place, they had long been cleared. Two sycamores stood some way behind the property, close to the main road rendered invisible by a drystone wall.

He lived in a bungalow that, from a distance, looked derelict. Thorn bushes and wild privet choked every reasonable approach but the front gate, with only a hint of a roof and skylight visible above this unruly line of vegetation.

The house wasn't the first thing Freya spotted. That was the boat, of course, a twenty-foot craft whose beige paintwork with brown trim dated it from some time in the 1980s, if not slightly earlier. It was called '*Contessa*', according to the lettering slashed along the side in what was presumably a facsimile of red lipstick. 'Eighties, then,' she mumbled to herself.

The boat was perched on top of a trailer missing its truck, parked in front of the house much as a car might be. If there was water anywhere nearby, Freya would have had to consult a map to find it.

A man emerged from below deck when she appeared. He wore a short-sleeved plaid shirt, turquoise shorts that gave the air surrounding them the tone of an optical illusion, and flip-flops. He was about average height, lean and well-muscled at the calves. His face contrasted with the lines of his body – it was bearded, in an attempt to hide red marks and blemishes that she saw creeping up his cheeks, even from a distance – the signal of a drinker, perhaps. Freya knew this from a lifetime's observations of some of the characters her mother served in the pub.

He said nothing when she approached, but viewed her frankly. A grin split his face, when it became clear Freya was not simply passing by. 'Well, someone's dressed for the weather,' he said. There was a touch of an Irish accent in there, but the voice seemed dusty, unused.

Freya ignored the jibe. 'Are you Mick Harvie?'

'Who wants to know?' The grin remained.

'My name's Freya Bain. I've come to you about a story I'm preparing for the national press. I was looking for your help.'

'I'm retired.'

'I know that. I think you'll be interested in my story, though. I need your help. You've got the contacts in the business, I've been told.'

'Most of them are dead, or retired. But they managed to find their sons and daughters jobs, I suppose. What's your story, Freya Bain?'

'It's about Gareth Solomon.'

Harvie said nothing. He wasn't grinning any more.

'You wrote the best book on the case. It's the bible, really, for anyone studying it. In fact, I went over it again on the train down here.' She pulled the book from her backpack – *Hunting the Woodcutter*.

'You want an autograph or something?' He wiped his hands on an old dishtowel, already discoloured with oil, and draped it over a rail. 'I can give you an autograph. No problem. But, unless you've found something linking that bastard to the missing people he's topped over the years, then I'm not really interested. I hope you haven't come a long way.'

'I don't have any new evidence as yet. Although I have been told he's preparing an appeal.'

'Course he is! He's always preparing an appeal. I bet he's been gibbering about some magical new evidence he's got, or some witness or other he's about to pull out of a hat, or his own suspect. I've heard it all before. To my face. He's lied so much about the people he killed he's started to believe it himself. This guy's a class-A liar, if nothing else. Look… I may not look it, but I am busy here. What's your story?'

'Gareth Solomon is my father.'

He wiped his hands again, reflexively, on the oily rag, as he sized Freya up. Then he clucked his tongue and said: 'How do you take your tea?'

The bungalow was tight-packed with a lifetime's belongings, but it wasn't untidy. Books and nautical ornaments crammed the available shelf-space across a number of wall units, but Freya had to admit she quite liked it. With its plain whitewashed walls offsetting the riot of the book spines, it had the feel of a university professor's office or a cosy den. An ornate marble fireplace completed the snug feel of the place, although there wasn't a speck of ash or any other hints that a fire had been lit there any time in the past year.

Freya blew onto the surface of a strong, thick cup of tea. Harvie sat in front of her in a battered but sturdy leather armchair with brass studs up and down the arms. 'When did you find out?' he asked.

'My mother told me. She's dead now.'

'Deathbed confession?' His eyes gleamed over the lip of his own cup as he took a drink.

'Not exactly. She hinted at telling me before she died – then put it in writing, for when the solicitor read out her will.'

'Dramatic enough, I guess. And is she quite sure it was him?'

'Seemed certain.'

'You do look like him. Or, you've got the same eyes, that's for sure. Difficult to tell with all that make-up. But I'll be candid with you – and I guess you're old enough to be wise – just because someone tells you who your father is, well… it doesn't necessarily mean they're your father.'

'I've given a DNA sample to his lawyer.'

'Who's that?' Harvie asked, sharply. 'Not Levison, is it? Blonde, big hair, looks like she starred in *Dallas*?'

'Yes, her name was Levison.'

'Hmm.' He clucked his tongue again. 'Can't decide if that's a smart move, or not. Probably not, knowing her.'

'She seemed a bit of a mess, to me. Looked like she'd

come back from a dirty stop-out. Looked about ready for another one, in fact.'

'Oh, don't swallow that act. I bet she pretended she was busy on her phone when she spoke with you. Or gibbered about how great the cocktails were.'

'She did seem kind of distracted, considering she'd set the meeting up.'

'Yep. Ding! That's what she does. Of course, if you're of the opposite sex, she's got other ways of throwing you off guard. Don't be fooled. Every great conjuror has that kind of act down to a fine art – they act the fool, or they pretend to be clumsy, or they start stuttering and telling bad jokes. It's all to deceive you. One hand starts waving, you should pay attention to what the other one's doing. She's got a lot of scalps on her mantelpiece, that one. Her front path is paved with the bones of people who underestimated her.'

'You have experience of this?'

'Oh yeah.' He snickered. 'You say she put you onto me?'

'Yes. Said you could help. Told me you had the contacts, and the knowledge.'

'I guess I do. I could make a couple of phone calls. But I'm wondering… what does Cheryl Levison get out of it? Or your dad, come to think of it?'

'She said the appeal is being heard. Takes time going through the courts. So I presume her putting me onto you has got something to do with that.'

'That's about right. You'll be useful to them. She'll have spotted that right away.' Harvie set down his cup, very delicately, then rested his head on his fist. 'I'll say this, it's unsettling.'

'What is?'

'The more I look at you, the more I see a resemblance. You've got those inky black eyes. They don't seem to reflect the light. He was like that. So you remind me of him… but you're also pretty. It's a bit like back in my courting days. I'd meet a girl I liked, and then find out she's the spitting image of her old man. Images you don't want in your mind, you know?'

'Excuse me?' She almost burst out laughing. But she was all too aware that she was with a strange man, in the strange man's house, in a very lonely spot.

'You're kind of Spanish-looking, if that's not too offensive a thing to say. Hispanic, that might be the term to use. That Goth stuff doesn't work on everyone, but it suits you down to the ground. You were made for mourning. I could see you fluttering a Sevillian fan in front of that pretty face.'

'Did we just time-warp fifty years into the past or something?'

He held out a placatory hand, but seemed unruffled for it. 'Just being honest with you. Old Fleet Street eye. I know what sells the papers. If they still sell papers. You take a nice picture, I'll bet.'

'Yeah, that's what I…'

'And that is what will sell your story. Everywhere.'

'I just want to write a piece. I'm not bothered about pictures.'

'If you want to be paid for it, properly, then you should be bothered about pictures. This isn't the time to get shy. If you give them a tip, and say: "Guess what? I'm the Woodcutter's daughter", then your face is going to appear in their papers whether you want it or not. Because they'll find you. They could be sat on a park bench half a mile away, but they'll get some pictures of you in the street. You would never know. Some joker might doorstep you, and you might even tell them to bugger off. But they'll get what they need out of you – and if not you, then your friends. And maybe even not your friends. Work colleagues, people you don't like. Exes. They might decide to take an unfriendly line of inquiry. It's more fun that way. For them, and the morons who read it. Then they'll run the story you wanted for yourself, except you had nothing to do with it, and you don't get a bean. They have ways of finding you. The dark arts, they call it. I'm a long time out the game, but that kind of stuff is easier to sort out in the digital era compared to what I worked with.'

Freya sighed. 'I'll have to think about that.'

'Suit yourself. I'm just telling you how it is. So what kind of piece are you aiming for, then? Magazine feature? "What it's like to have a dad who's a murderer"?'

'No. The opposite. One for the news section.'

'Yeah? What's your angle?'

'I don't think he did it.'

'You what?' Now it was Harvie's turn for incredulity. 'He's a killer, love. Don't doubt it. I worked on a few serial killer cases. They were much more common in the Eighties and Nineties than they are now, with a camera on every bloody corner. Much harder for them to get away with it, these days. With the really bad ones, you get to know them. You can separate the truth from the lies. And I know your dad's a killer. Many times over. Bet your life on it.'

'He told me he didn't do it. Seemed sure. I guess I believed him.'

Harvie openly barked laughter. He had ugly teeth, Freya

saw, chipped like old crockery. 'No offence. I know this is a weird time for you. You said your mother died quite recently, is that right? OK – it's a stressful business all round. And out of the blue, this father figure appears. And he's got this amazing story about how he got fitted up for something he didn't do. Don't give it headspace. Gareth Solomon is a liar. It's part of his make-up. Hopefully not genetic, for your sake. He won't take responsibility for anything, because he has no empathy. People are there to be manipulated. You know what he did, right? You know how he did it?'

'I've read your book.'

'He captured people, let them loose in remote places – confined environments – caught up with them before they could escape, and chopped them to pieces. That's what he did.'

'He was convicted of one murder, and that was on circumstantial evidence. And there was nothing physical linking him to June Caton-Bell.'

'There's plenty of circumstantial evidence linking him to every case connected to the Woodcutter. Times, places, the jobs he was doing, his knowledge of the areas. All that's missing are the bodies and the witnesses.'

Freya swallowed. 'How about the woman who escaped? Natalie Grey? She spoke about a completely different man.'

'Natalie Grey got bashed over the head for her trouble, and I know from meeting her more than once over the years, she's still not right. Suggestion of brain damage, added to a whole textbook's worth of psychological trauma. It's something that happened with one or two people who got away from the Yorkshire Ripper, and others. They got confused in the heat of the moment – entirely understandably.

And their experiences scarred them for life. Natalie Grey is a lovely woman, and my heart's broken for her, but... No.'

'That stance could support either theory,' Freya said, smartly. 'That he's either the killer, or he's been fitted up by Bernard Galvin and the rest of his team on the Woodcutter inquiry.'

Mick Harvie pinched his eyebrows. 'Bernard Galvin... and you can write this down if you like, a direct quote... is one of the biggest arseholes I've ever met in my life. But he's also one of the best coppers. And he wasn't bent. Never in his life. I take offence at that on his behalf. I'm no fan of Bernie, far less a friend. I felt the rough side of his tongue more than once. But he's a straight shooter. And the Woodcutter inquiry almost killed him. He had a heart attack, and his own top men didn't even know. And it haunts him that he couldn't pin the other murders on Solomon. Especially in light of the fact the bodies are missing. I know that. Even now, he's out there, looking for the other bodies. He might never find them. But he got his man. I know that for sure. I don't like him, but I respect him. So, I'll ask you kindly – never run him down in front of me.'

'Noted,' Freya said.

'Now... seeing as I know what your angle is – what's the hook?'

She smiled. 'That would be telling.'

'So – that means you've got something new?'

'Oh, I'm just here to take a nice picture. Don't you mind what I know or not. What would I know?'

He grinned. 'Touché, miss. But if you want my help, you'll have to do better than that. What's in it for me?'

'I'll give your book a plug. I'll even give you a quote.'

He laughed aloud. 'You've got the gumption, that's for sure! You might do all right in this game.'

'You might have to rewrite it. If I prove that my father's not the Woodcutter.'

'It'd be big news, there's no denying that. I'll set something up for you. You're on.'

'Shake on it?'

He did – but after he'd let Freya's hand go, his demeanour changed. 'I've got something I want to show you. It might end up getting me in trouble. But I think it's worth it, in this case. Wait here a minute.'

Freya sat in the silence, growing oddly apprehensive. When Mick Harvie returned, he was carrying an old ring binder. Inside it were clear plastic wallets. He flicked through the files, then stopped at one in particular. He took care to take out what was inside – a black and white photograph. He held it by the corner, as if it was only just developed, and turned it towards Freya.

'I obtained these from a friend on the force. I'm not supposed to have them. I was pushing for it to be published in the book alongside the other stills, but... taste and decency, and all that. It might not be totally clear what you're looking at, here,' Harvie said. 'You need to look closely. Up at the top...'

'I can see it,' Freya said, her voice almost a whisper. 'There's a head.'

'Nope, not a head. Not intact, anyway. But you can see eyes. He made sure Caton-Bell's eyes were open. He wanted people to discover her; that's the thing. He was taking more of a risk. Because I can tell you this about the Woodcutter: he was getting a taste for it. He was a thrill killer. But just kidnapping and hunting people in the woods wasn't doing it for him any more. He needed a greater risk of getting caught. Now when you next look into your daddy dearest's eyes, you think about these eyes. What you are looking at is what used to be a person. He kidnapped her, took her into the middle of a forest, then hunted her in the dead of night. But someone saw him. Someone who picked him out of an ID parade. Now I want you to remember this: no matter what your father says to you, he did this. He chopped a twenty-seven-year-old paramedic and part-time club bouncer in the prime of her life into pieces. Then he chopped some of the pieces into more pieces.'

'Put that away. That does nothing for what I've said.' She sniffed; she was hardly aware she'd been crying, until tears ran off her chin and pattered onto her skirt.

Harvie's expression softened. He appeared shocked that she had been in tears. 'I'm sorry, love. I didn't do that just to shock you. I did it to shake you out of any idea that your dad's worth listening to. The guy who did that – he's not normal, and he's not nice. No matter how much you want him to be. You want to work with me, bear that in mind.'

'I think I'd better go. I'll leave you my number – let me know if your contacts pay off. Tell them I want to speak to them, and I want to be paid for an exclusive. I'm sure you'll get some tip money for it.'

Harvie slid the photograph back into its wallet. 'OK. You're on.'

8

It went against her nature so much it felt like a nightmare. Reality given a near-perverse twist; the shock of exposure, of being front and centre, of drawing the eye. This had never been Freya. But it was necessary. Harvie had been persuasive. He'd been up-front about the benefits to this farce, this public display that was the polar opposite of how Freya usually conducted herself. This was something she had to do, he'd said, in order to get to the truth. And also in order to give herself a future. He'd said this would give her a start in the business. He mentioned all kinds of future scenarios, even a life in front of a camera. "Play your cards right, you could front documentaries. You could explore other people's stories, similar to yours." All along, this was underpinned by his insistence that Gareth Solomon was a killer, and that Freya was another type of victim.

Freya wanted to believe her father, which she knew was a failing. But quite detached from this, her reason told her that he had a case.

The shoot was part of the deal, set up by Harvie. She felt so awkward that Harvie offered her a drink from a hip flask she'd never noticed him carrying before. She refused.

The photographer made her part her fringe. He actually used his fingers to do it, flicking it back over her ears. 'Sorry, love – you want to be in this article, or not?'

Freya took a step back, defensively. It was the 'love' as much as the hands. 'I didn't know you were a fashion consultant.'

'Could be doing with a bit less make-up around the eyes, too. It does look brilliant – but we have to see those eyes. You've got your father's eyes, for sure – that's the big sell. Put images of the two of you together and...' He snapped his fingers and grinned.

The photographer looked and sounded much older than he was – blond, stout and thick-lipped, the kind of overgrown baby you dreaded to see take root in your favourite pub. He wasn't wearing off-grey jogging bottoms, but it was easy to picture him doing so.

'You can see my eyes just fine. It's make-up, not sunglasses.'

'I've got some wet wipes in the car...'

'Whatever for?'

In the background, resting against a fence, Mick Harvie snorted, and turned his head away.

'For people who need their noses wiped before we do a shoot,' the photographer said, sullenly.

'I'm sorry,' Freya said, diffidently. 'I've chosen this look for a reason. I'm going with it.'

'It's just that, you look... Well, you look scary. Proper scare-the-kids scary. I mean, it's up to you, it's your decision.'

'That's right. It is,' Freya said evenly.

'She won't always have the dark eye make-up on, or the whiter-than-white face,' Harvie said. 'Isn't that right? I'd put money on you being in disguise, if I was a betting man. Which I am.'

Freya smiled. 'Spot on. There are too many nutters out there. They see me in a paper or on a website, fine. They won't link it to me in real life. Who knows... I might wear a different shade of black.'

Harvie grinned. The photographer shrugged, and checked his outsized camera. It was more of a bazooka, something that should have been rested on someone else's shoulder. 'OK,' he said. 'We'll do some of you next to the forest, with it over your shoulder, then some of you in the foreground. Then maybe we'll head inside.' He turned to Harvie. 'You know the spot, right?'

Harvie nodded. 'It's a little way in. Off the beaten path. They grew trees in the spot where he caught her, though. Planted them about a year and a bit later. Thick vegetation all around it. Brambles. Thorns. Quite a good idea. Let Mother Nature obliterate a nasty patch. It also stops the weirdos. Of which there are many. You know – people who want to come in and pose for pictures.'

'Can't legislate for them, Mick.' All Freya could see was the photographer's uneven grin as he put the camera to his eye. 'All right. Let's do a few now, loosen you up a bit, love... It's OK, keep your hands clasped for now. Maybe turn a little to the left, get you in profile... Lovely, you've got an excellent jawline – that works really well.'

She tried to ignore the treacherous feelings his flatteries and mild exhortations had on her and simply followed instructions. She even smiled once or twice – a sad smile, she knew. The only one she had. She kept her eye on the waving line of trees that marked the start of Elsingham Forest, a green space on the fringes of a new town in the Midlands, whose unpleasant sprawl of pylons, shopping centres and pockets of red-brick houses was visible to the south. The forest was an oasis, and was meant to be – threaded through with paths for mountain bikers as well as a network of walking or running routes stretching out for twenty-one K in total. It was here that the killer dubbed the Woodcutter by none other than Mick Harvie had claimed his final victim. He had left the body to be discovered in a clearing, after taking June Caton-Bell into the woods after dark, after she had been abducted while walking her dog down a lonely road sixty miles away.

Forensic analysis of the disturbed vegetation had shown that a desperate chase had taken place. Some of the marks on the body parts indicated that she had run through thick vegetation, and on one occasion had even tried to hide under a rotten tree. Whatever she'd tried, it hadn't worked. The Woodcutter caught up with her, and it was here he'd lived up to his name.

Sometimes when Freya closed her eyes, she could see Mick Harvie's black and white pictures of the body. A gory pile that didn't look like a body at all, until you looked closely. Which was exactly what the person who'd found the body – another luckless dog walker – had done, early in the morning, less than three hours after the Woodcutter had chopped it up with a fire axe.

It was the only body to be found in the case; but there were four more very similar abductions, dating around the same time. Four women and a man, all young and fit.

There was no obvious sexual element to what had been done to June Caton-Bell. The thrill, or so the thinking went, came from the hunt.

But it was here that the Woodcutter, so they said, had made his cardinal error. It had been high summer, and there was plenty of light in the sky by the time a man had been seen by a woman who owned a cottage on the fringes of the woods. A keen birdwatcher, the woman had a pair of binoculars to hand, and had seen a man with dark hair and a large military-style backpack. She had a glimpse of his face – enough to pick him out of a police line-up later, once the slow snare of police work pinpointed a drifter named Gareth Solomon who had been working as a delivery driver at the time.

Once the photographer had finished for the day and left for a job in the afternoon featuring a senior member of the royal family opening a petting zoo about twenty miles away, Mick Harvie walked Freya back to his car.

'I had a look at your feature,' he said. 'Needs a bit of work. But quite a good effort.'

'Thanks. Did you pass it on to Nuala Franklin? She's the features editor, I think.'

'Oh yeah. I remember Nuala, in fact; though she claims not to remember me. I still see a kid fresh out of college, but I guess she's about forty now. Anyway, yeah, she's well on board. But I know exactly what she's going to say.'

'And that is...?'

'You need to state an opinion on your dad. And state it clearly.'

'I don't have one. I've met him once.'

'Really?' Harvie grinned. 'Not sure I believe that.'

'Believe what you like.'

'Yeah… you describe him well. A touch melodramatic, but it is a little bit dramatic to meet your dad, the serial killer. Very Hannibal Lecter and Clarice. Like it.'

'I just described what he said and what he looked like. I wasn't writing a novel about it.'

'What we don't get is… your gut feeling. Do you think he did it? I think people need to know that.'

'I can't know if he did it. It's not certain. So I can't say if I don't know.'

'I'm not talking about knowledge. I'm talking about *feeling*. You don't have to quote the science behind it, or show your working.'

'I just don't know. It'd be different if he'd been in my life – like a normal father. Do you have any kids, Mick?'

He didn't answer that, but he said: 'Let's put it another way. If I had to put a gun to your head, what's your feeling?'

'My feeling is no. He didn't do it.'

Harvie laughed. 'You're serious?'

'Yes. There it is. You asked. That's my answer. I don't think he's guilty. I believed him. But I'll admit… there's something off about the guy. No doubting that. I didn't feel *comfortable*. But that could be something to do with the high-security prison, or the guards. Or the context. Or the possibility that he might have chopped five people up, for a laugh, whatever he says.'

Harvie nodded. 'That's the right answer. I'll drive you all the way home, if you like. You let me know if the cash arrives – should be in your account today from the paper. They work fast, these days. Instant transfer. Readies on demand. Used to be, you were waiting on the postie bringing a cheque.'

'It's there already, in fact.'

'There you go.'

Before she got in the car, Freya took once last look at the treeline, a blackened crucible stretching out for a couple of miles in either direction. A father and two young children emerged from one of the paths. One of the youngsters was on a bike with stabilisers, cheering at the sudden open path and the increased speed. Freya shivered, and got into Harvie's car.

9

She settled down back at the flat, clicking off the television and opening the laptop at the kitchen table. It had been a while since Freya had had to take notes, and arrange them into something that made sense. School had been a long time ago, now, and she'd never gone to university or college. At first, she'd bridled at the information that appeared on her screen about the Woodcutter. There had been reports over the years – some detailing violent incidents Gareth Solomon had been involved in, some as victim, but just as often as perpetrator. She tried to connect that sort of life, that feral existence behind bars, with her own, and couldn't. Although she'd dealt with many strange and nasty customers when she'd worked behind the bar with her mother, she could not visualise what it must be like to exist in jail, to pull a man's leg clean out of its socket, as one report claimed he had done. They used a particular photo to illustrate this story, and it was one that Freya had grown accustomed to – Gareth Solomon, teeth bared, his composure surrendered, running the gauntlet of photographers outside court as he made his way to the prison van after his trial. No blanket draped over the head for Gareth Solomon; they'd simply escorted him out, turning him into something of a show pony.

His almost canine leer, lips peeled back, black eyes reflecting a photographer's flashbulb in searing white crescents, was difficult to look at for too long.

Freya became aware that she had her back to an open door. She closed it, then turned the machine around and sat at the other side of the table, her back to the wall.

Opening a text document, Freya began to note down dates and times. She kept bumping into one website in particular, one that was professionally laid out compared to many of the others she looked at, although the prose could be a little flowery. Red Ink, it was called. While some of the murder websites had an obvious relish for the grotesque and the skin-crawling detail of crime scene photos, Red Ink was sober, and gave clear warnings when objectionable content was about to appear.

It also had a clear timeline, from which she cribbed the majority of her notes.

First victim: Anne-Marie Kittrick.

There was a picture of a girl with natural dirty blonde hair and bright red lipstick – she was out at a party. The analogue shot was slightly blurry, as if there were flames at the bottom of the screen, and she was clearly on a night out. Her top was plated gold, and her arms were bare. They were the arms of someone with little fat on their bones, and her neck and shoulders hinted at a swimmer. Anne-Marie was twenty-two years old when she vanished on a training run for a half-marathon, in the summer of 1994. Her route had taken her over a cattle grid and into an underpass – photographed in all its terrifying detail on Red Ink. It was the type of place Freya would have instinctively ignored, even as a person who routinely ran down alleyways and in quieter forest paths. It was a place a troll might have lived; it was where Anne-Marie was abducted.

Whoever had done it was efficient and cunning, possibly having parked at a rest area just off the main road above, a place hidden by the trees in full leaf at the height of summer. He had taken a chance on being the only vehicle present in the lay-by, and the gamble had paid off. There were signs of a brief struggle, but little or no physical evidence to go on, and no body, either. Anne-Marie had just had her graduation ceremony, and was preparing to do a master's after the summer. The half-marathon had been scheduled for that September, and she had been confident of a good time.

Second victim: Coleen Arden.

Coleen Arden was a beautiful girl who had been a catalogue model in her Edinburgh childhood. She had settled down south. When she vanished she was twenty-four years old and working as a paralegal. She had varied interests including horse-riding and, latterly, canoeing. Coleen had a habit of taking a train every Saturday out into the South Downs, in order to climb a six-hundred-foot hill. The significance of this baffled her friends, who often implored her to stay out on a Friday night with them, but it seemed to be an unshakable commitment when she had spare time. It was rumoured that the hill was a similar physical challenge to climbing Arthur's Seat, a weekly ritual with her father when she was growing up. It was almost certainly this ritual that brought her into contact with the Woodcutter. She vanished without trace in October 1994, on a bleak, wet day.

Coleen left haunting images on prototype CCTV, caught on videotape at a shop as she walked to the train station, a slender, tall figure in expensive hiking gear and waterproof clothing, chin held high, on her way to the train. Freya thought she looked like someone who had once been on *Coronation Street*, a strikingly attractive girl.

Freya typed a quick note: Not party girls?

Victim three: Max Dilworth.

Max Dilworth was the outlier. There were many theories that Dilworth had met his end at the hands of someone else in February 1995, but how he had vanished matched the MO of the Woodcutter. He was a former squaddie, twenty-seven years old, having done five years with the Royal Artillery. He was working as a security guard for the time being but had plans to join the prison service. He had kept up his excellent physical fitness, combining running with weight training – a formidable-looking young man with sharp, even chiselled features. 'Ladies' man', said the profile on Red Ink, somewhat acidly. Max Dilworth had disappeared off a canal track. Tyre tracks spotted near a rest area usually filled by a mobile coffee stand had matched a transit van, stolen years before, which was later found burnt out. This was the closest investigators came to obtaining a physical clue in these cases.

Victim four: Danielle Pearson.

Danielle was a swimmer who had been out walking her dog down a country lane during the Easter holidays in 1995. An eighteen-year-old first-year student, tall, red-haired and pale-skinned, with a delicate starfield of freckles across her cheeks, she was the youngest of the Woodcutter's victims. She had been home for the holidays and enjoying a nice walk on a clear, cool evening across an old railway track, fringed with wheatfields. There were no signs of a struggle, but there must have been one: the dog, a fairly handy German shepherd named Bo, was found with its skull cleft in two. An axe had been used to kill the dog, and it had taken one single, savage blow to do it.

Victim five: June Caton-Bell.

This was how they had caught him. June Caton-Bell had disappeared after working on the doors of a nightclub in a small Essex town, the only such place for miles around, serving people who came in from dozens of towns nearby. As such, it was not in want of any action, and June Caton-Bell was known as someone who could handle herself, easily a match for the men who caused trouble as well as the women. An experienced and intuitive bouncer, she was well regarded by colleagues and trained at a local boxing club alongside the men. But she wasn't quite the hard case she seemed; she had been training to become a paramedic, and she had been regarded as a promising student who had a passion for helping people.

June Caton-Bell had walked home in the early hours of

the morning after a shift, skirting a massive country park, which had a reputation for its ancient forest. It was here that she was chased down and chopped up, with her body discovered hours later. This case could also be regarded as an outlier because the body had been discovered, whereas in the other four cases, remains had yet to be recovered. It was here that a man with dark hair and eyes was seen getting into a black transit van, not long after June Caton-Bell was estimated to have died, by the woman who lived in a tiny cottage, partly hidden from the main road. The woman used her birdwatcher's eye to identify the man in a subsequent ID parade as Gareth Solomon, a long-distance driver who was known to have been passing the area at the time. Solomon had been convicted of killing Caton-Bell, on very flimsy circumstantial evidence.

There were theories that the Woodcutter was behind other abductions, the most compelling case involving a Dutch backpacker called Florence Ceulemans, who had disappeared while she had been working on a farm in the summer of 1994. No one had ever been arrested over her death, although the rural setting, and the girl's slender, tall physique and high level of physical fitness fit the profile of the Woodcutter's victims.

One woman had escaped: Natalie Grey, the woman Harvie had spoken of, who had been snatched off the street but had fought hard to avoid being put into a dark van. She had been beaten savagely over the head when someone came to help and she'd managed to scream, and was left for dead at the roadside. She had suffered head injuries that led to lasting damage. Her memory of the event was understandably but annoyingly hazy. She had mentioned a dark van and a man with black hair and eyes – although she had also mentioned a beard, which her father did not have at that point.

Freya hit the final full stop, then sat back, staring at the document. That was it – the five victims, plus one who was possibly abducted and one woman who had escaped.

Now it was time to ask her dad about them.

10

The man the world knew as the Woodcutter clapped his hands with some glee as his daughter sat down in front of him in the visitors' room.

'This is like Christmas! Twice in a matter of weeks! Usually hardly anyone comes to see me. Psychologists wanting to write about serial killers in their PhDs, for the most part. Or journalists. I've learned not to speak to them, over the years. The psychologists are the worst.'

Freya was startled by how animated he got, how child-like he seemed in his enthusiasm. She wondered if she would ever feel relaxed in his presence, even if there was a pane of glass separating them and some bulky, stern men to act as an extra bulwark, if necessary.

This is going to take some getting used to. That'd be true even if he wasn't in jail for being a maniac.

'Speaking of journalists... how about Mick Harvie?' she asked.

'Harvie... You met him? How's he looking these days?'

'Little wiry bloke, crooked teeth? Looks like he's been sleeping in a skip for the night.'

'That's uncannily close to how he looked years ago,' Solomon said. 'I used to speak to him a fair bit...'

'He expected you to be a bit more forthcoming?'

'Well, no. He expected me to be *guilty*. He expected me to admit it, to maybe look for the notoriety or something. He soon got bored of me denying everything and asking him to set the record straight. You don't sell too many books by taking that angle. Or maybe I've just got one of those guilty faces. So, he spoke to just about everyone else. My miserable family. He missed you, though. It must have irritated him to realise that.'

'For all I know, he's writing a sequel.'

Solomon raised an eyebrow. 'And what are you writing?'

'Me? Well, I'm writing some articles. I want to get to the truth of what happened. That's where you can help me.'

'My appeal is ongoing. Can't say too much about it. Can't prejudice a supreme court judge and all that, but quietest is safest.' He sighed. 'Sorry about that. You look disappointed. This is the first time I've properly disappointed my daughter. I'm going to have to take a minute or two to process it.'

'I don't mean about your appeal. Not as such.' Freya cleared her throat. He had a way of staring that made her uncomfortable. He didn't blink or break eye contact. It seemed to be some kind of intimidatory tactic – perhaps it was second nature behind bars – and she had to admit, it worked well. 'I mean about you. I mean about your life.'

'Biography, then. Got you.' He winked.

'No. I'm curious. It's not for a book. It's not for a project. It doesn't even have to be about why you're in here. It's about you.'

'Say again?'

'I want to know about my dad. It's not for an article. It's not for homework. It isn't for a book report. You're my dad.' Her voice faltered; she surprised herself with the emotion that bubbled out, just for a second.

Solomon almost looked angry at this, but his tone was gentle when he spoke. 'What is it you want to know?'

'Where are you from?'

'I'm a Yorkshireman. Born in Bradford. If you want to pinpoint a place I came from, you could say it's there. I was in care for a while. So, well, that was fun. Schooling didn't amount to much in that environment. The subjects I enjoyed most were art, technical studies, craft and design – working with your hands, really.'

'I want to know about family. Where you come from. What were my grandparents like?'

'Well, Mummy ran off, which I suppose was a formative experience. That was when I was four. I can barely remember her. Dark eyes. Like me. Like you. She already had three kids, two girls and a boy, not much older than me. I can't recall them too much, either. Her maiden name was Lawrence. Sally Lawrence. I remember a wedding portrait of them. Late fifties. They must have loved each other. Anyway, David Solomon, builder by trade, struggled a little bit with us young ones. But he had his outlets – drinking, fish and chips on a Friday, and a good supply of tarts... Sorry. That language isn't any good any more. A stream of young ladies, who would sometimes stay the night. I slept in the bedroom next to his, and had to listen to them. Had a bit of stamina, your grandad – I'll say that for him. Anyway, that aside, his other hobbies were beating the shit out of us, and me in particular.'

He took a sip of water from a plastic cup; the eyes of both guards fixed on him intently as he did so.

'I looked more like her than my brothers and sisters – which is to say I looked nothing like him. He raised this quite a lot, you know – "You aren't mine", he would say. He broke the crowns off my front teeth with one single punch. A cracker, I have to say. He had a good dig on him. Thankfully they were just baby teeth. Anyway, after that, the school got involved, and the rest of the kids were taken into care. I lost contact… Someone once told me he died. Sally is dead as well.'

'You lost contact with your siblings?'

'Yeah. They're easy enough to look up – Mick Harvie took the liberty of doing it for me. None of them had much good to say about me. Roger, my elder brother, told some absolute lies. Stuff about me torturing animals, that kind of thing. We threw rocks at rats down the back of the Scout hall, I'll admit to that, but the rest of it was bollocks. That's the thing about being convicted of murder, even if it's one you didn't do – it makes it very hard for you to sue people for libel.'

He grinned at this, delighted with the witticism. He was growing louder, as if warming to his theme. Either he was someone who couldn't shut up during normal times, or he was someone who didn't speak at all, and had finally been given an outlet.

'Next up was the children's home. That's where I got my first taste of sexual abuse, on top of the physical. A music teacher, would you believe, a Mr Umber – never forget the name. And you know, some days I was grateful for the affection.' He barked laughter, but no one else did.

Freya's shoulders bunched tight, as if a hand had seized her by the scruff of the neck. 'That's awful. How can you laugh about it?'

'Well, as I've always said – people will joke about stuff. It's part of being human. Even if you're not quite human. Tell someone they're going to hell, chances are they'll joke about it. Even when they're staring the devil right in the eyes.'

'You need therapy. You need to talk to someone. Not just me.'

'I've talked to a bunch of psychologists. As I told you – they're the worst. Although I enjoy trying to get a smile out of them.'

'Did you ever go to the police?'

'God, no. You accepted it as part and parcel of the school experience. You got treats in return – sweets and crisps, and then beer, as we got older. It seemed an acceptable trade-off. Someone grassed on him, though. They found him hanging in a shed at his house. Married, wife, kids, would you believe. I think it all came out. There was an inquiry after it. I was never called as a witness. Anyway, from there, I fell into the wonderful world of work, with Mrs Thatcher's revolution in full swing. I worked at a warehouse, packing clothes for a catalogue company. There, I made the sanest, most practical decision of my life. I learned to drive, then got an HGV licence. I didn't like it on the big wagons, so I drove a van, worked as a courier, taking packages and transferring parts to garages, that kind of stuff. I even transported dodgier things, no questions asked. It was great money. I moved around a lot. And that's probably where the final psychological piece of the puzzle falls into place. I must admit, I do tick a lot of those serial killer boxes.'

'How about friends? Girlfriends?'

He shrugged. 'I had some, here and there. But they never lasted. Life wasn't built for friends.'

Freya felt a tingle of recognition. She thought of the empty flat; her empty bed.

'I felt I was in shock, a lot of my life. I lived with blame. A psychologist might tell you that I felt guilt – guilt at my mother having left; guilt at my dad for blaming me for it; guilt that I didn't stop the abuse. Thing is, though… I can't tell you whether guilt is real for me, or not. But I've found it hard to get friends. Bit of a loner, maybe. But women… I worked out how to get those.'

'Tell me about them.'

Solomon bit the inside of his mouth. 'Nah, that's enough about me. Now – tell me about you.'

'What do you mean?'

'The same. I've told you my life story – now tell me yours.'

'Well… there's not much to tell.'

'There is. Of course there is. Tell me about Mary. Tell me about your mum.' He crossed his legs and linked his hands over one knee. Freya could not tell if his expression of sincerity was a dreadful fake, or too intense for comfort. She didn't like it either way.

'Well… I stayed in the town. You know. Where you and Mary met.' Freya cleared her throat. 'I didn't have any siblings, and Mum was a care home kid herself.'

Solomon's eyes widened. 'That's right! She was! I remember now. I think we bonded over that. Both kids in care. What do you know?' He seemed delighted at the memory.

'So, it was just me and her. She went back to work in the pub. A lot of the time I was left with a woman I remember as Auntie Lesley, but she wasn't a relation. House full of kids, a year between each sibling. I forget if there were eight or nine of them... It didn't bring me out of my shell. I was quiet. Mary always told me I was quiet. I think I believed her. I had some friends at primary school, but no best friends. I was invited to parties, but couldn't gel with kids my own age. I was... the word is weird. It's not a nice word. But it's me.' Freya noticed the prison officers staring at her, and cleared her throat, suddenly hesitant.

'Don't mind these gorillas. They've got hearts of gold, underneath that fleshy exterior.' Solomon was camp as Liberace as he said this, and grinned at one of them. The man looked away from her father abruptly.

'I think primary school was happy, for all that. I was drawn into my own worlds.'

'Tell me about Mary.'

'She was lovely. No-nonsense. Sense of an Irish mammy. Wicked sense of humour. Lots of fun. Lots of friends. Brought some of them back from the pub after closing time. She loved a sing-song, but it was never a bad crowd, never bad people.'

'Were there ever any uncles for you to get to know?' Solomon asked quietly. 'Or step-dads, if you want a less quaint term?'

'Some... No one who came to live with us. We were a team, really. It wouldn't be fair to say we were like sisters, but I was very close to her. Clingy, even. And she worried about me all the time. My idea of a great night was being sat with her, watching *The X Factor* with a hot chocolate.'

'Homebody,' he mused. 'That's sweet. Part of me thinks I would have liked to have been a homebody. I feel a little tug in my heart when I think about that, you know? A little nip.

A nice, safe, warm family home. Christmases, even. What were Christmases like?'

'You'll have to unwrap that later,' the guard nearest Freya said, tapping his watch. 'Your time's up.'

'I haven't even asked you about the case. The victims…' She was flustered, her face glowing.

'I don't know anything about any victims,' Solomon said, in a bored tone.

'I know, I mean… I'll… I'll come back,' Freya said, snatching up her notebook. 'We'll talk this over.'

'Oh, we will,' Solomon said, grinning. 'This has been enjoyable. Even stranger, it's been… *interesting*.'

11

In order to escape the pinging phone and the creeping notifications across social media, Freya got on with dyeing her hair. The smell of the dye reminded her of her mother – she'd gone through a phase of having blackcurranty red through her hair, which had lasted until Freya had asked outright if it was Autumn Plum, and streaks of the stuff had lingered in the bathroom sink for a long time afterwards.

Freya took a good while to work up the courage to look at her handiwork, unwrapping it slowly. The colour didn't suit her eyes, she saw that right away, but it would do for now.

She was on the front cover of two newspapers. She put them face-downwards on the kitchen table, not minded to pick them up again. One saving grace: she had taken a lovely photograph, at least in the newspaper where she'd sold her story.

Mick Harvie had screwed her over, of course. She'd had the byline in the *Salvo* – that had all been above board. But he'd also written his own piece, under his own name, in the tabloid's biggest rival. No professional photographs had accompanied that one, but the paper had ruthlessly plundered her social media profiles for other ones. She'd even been disgusted to note that pictures from last Christmas night out – the one where she'd kissed her little officemate – had also appeared. Either stolen or sold.

The article had been excruciating in its appraisal. To see ourselves as others see us, she thought, as she forced herself to read the article headlined: THE WOODCUTTER'S DAUGHTER. In the strapline underneath: Serial killer Gareth Solomon's secret daughter says: My father may not have done it.

The story had called her a 'diffident twenty-five-year-old, strikingly but strangely dressed, fond of thick eyeshadow and mascara, of the type you might recognise as a goth'. And it went on to say: 'She admits to a fascination for the dark side of life – particularly that of her father. Gareth Solomon was jailed for life eleven years ago for the murder of June Caton-Bell, but is suspected of having murdered at least four more young people who vanished without trace in suspiciously similar circumstances. Today, veteran investigative reporter Mick Harvie lifts the lid on the case that chilled the nation and dares to ask: was Gareth Solomon wrongly convicted?'

'Not what you said to me,' Freya huffed. 'Defended that dodgy copper to the hilt, didn't you?'

Then came the part that caused Freya to stand bolt upright, in the silent flat.

'I can exclusively reveal that the testimony that ultimately put Gareth Solomon in jail never made it to open court. Solomon had an alibi on the night June Caton-Bell was butchered in the forest all those years ago. He was having an affair with one of the investigating officers.'

Inset was a grainy picture – not taken all that long ago,

but weathered, pre-digital, sometime in the late 1990s going by the woman's blood-bright lipstick and powder-pale face. Her hair was black, and caught the light beautifully. She was pretty in a severe way – teacher-pretty – with big, heavy cheekbones that reminded Freya, disconcertingly, of her mother's features. The pic ID'd her as PC Carol Ramirez.

'When I contacted Ms Ramirez – who left the police soon after the conclusion of the Woodcutter case – she refused to comment on the matter. Nor did the police force who employed her.'

'How the hell did he find that out?' Freya yelped. She turned on her phone, scrolling past unacknowledged messages from her friends.

'What's the deal?' she asked Harvie, by text. 'PC Ramirez? Why didn't you tell me?'

He replied soon after. 'I'm a journalist.' Then he added an emoji depicting an animated figure shrugging its shoulders. 'And I kept up my end of the bargain. You've also got the contacts. You'll learn not to cry over spilt milk. You got a very good deal out of me. I'm not always so generous.' The message ended with a smiley emoji.

Freya had written and deleted several ripostes to this, before degenerating into angry, clenched-fist tears.

Still there had been offers from several newspapers, who had all somehow tracked her down. Text messages asking for interviews, including one from broadcast news.

It was all a mistake. I should have ignored this guy.

There she was, yet again, on the front page of the *Salvo*. Hand on her hip – not a good pose, really, although she looked thinner than she realised – with the jointed shadows of the woods over her shoulder. She was smiling, if only slightly. It was a face Freya might have wanted to slap, all things considered.

Then came an intriguing message on email. It was marked RInk.

> 'I have information regarding your father. He may have been the victim of a miscarriage of justice. Please don't delete this. First of all, visit www.crossedoutwithredink.co.uk My name's Glenn. I can help. Get in touch via the website – or give me a call.'

Freya clicked on the link; it took her through to a blog on what appeared to be famous murders, from Jack the Ripper through to some 'recent disappearances', decorated with mockingly jolly pictures of the dead or missing – people at Christmas parties, or in wedding outfits, or posing on beaches, or pouting for all they were worth on selfies. The top item on the blog bore her father's face as a masthead image – all the more striking for having been clumsily cropped. His eyes were freakishly insulated from light, as dark as they came. Like hers. It wasn't quite a malevolent stare, in his final mugshot, but it was unsettling, even for Freya. In a staring contest, you would have blinked first, gladly.

MISCARRIAGES OF JUSTICE – WAS THE WOODCUTTER SET UP?

There then followed a detailed, euphuistic blog, with paragraph stops and indeed full stops a rare respite from the dense text. It had appeared in her research into the victims earlier; she recalled the layout, now that she scrolled over it at her leisure.

One or two familiar pictures appeared: the luckless June Caton-Bell – pictured in rude health rather than a pile of sliced meat – the other victims, the police officer, and then Carol Ramirez – a different image, in full uniform, a big-hipped, heavy-breasted woman in a dress shirt. She looked more obviously Hispanic in this picture. She was the type of woman who might have been better suited as a prison officer, Freya thought, unkindly.

Freya read the blog for a while, then, before she could change her mind, she filled in the contact box.

'This is Freya. I got your text message. Very interested in how you managed to get my number. Anyway. Do let me know what information you have regarding my father.'

She wanted to add '...THE WOODCUTTER', all caps intended. Then realised that of all the missteps she'd made in the past few weeks, tormenting someone she didn't know on the internet had to be up there with the worst of them.

Freya hit send. Then she tore off the towel and stared at her hair. She mussed it up, ran a brush through it, then her expression softened in the mirror. Not bad. Might need a spot of spray to give it the ringlets look – but not bad at all. It didn't quite suit her – only black suited her eyes; this was a truism for Freya on a par with the earth being round, or water being wet – but it was striking.

'Yeah. Cover girl,' she said, wryly.

Freya turned away from the mirror, snatched up her keys, put on her jacket, and headed out into the street.

It wasn't long before she reached the lane down the back of the bigger houses, away from the Victorian block of flats where her mother had invested wisely, and carried on past an overgrown wooded area towards the farmer's fields. The sun had only just began to sink on the day she went nationwide with the story of who her father was; she'd secured another feature for the *Salvo*, this one on her impressions of her father at their first meeting – one she had still to write, ahead of the Saturday magazine. And she had something to go on: the possibility that he wasn't a killer, after all.

Freya made her way onto a track that cut through a field of cabbages, rutted where a tractor had passed only recently. Past the vegetation, there was a fenced-off housing estate, partly obscured by electricity pylons. Freya often walked out here, but never quite so late; you met the odd dog walker, but by and large the place was quiet, a public footpath that people didn't take owing to the local farmer's habit of discharging his guns, unseen. It was a secret place; Freya liked to go there to stretch her legs. She pulled her jacket close, and smiled.

Push through. Take deeper breaths. Get that lovely oxygen in. Let it fight off the acid build-up in your muscles, the sneering traitor that tells you to stop. Don't bounce on your heels. Don't fight gravity. Don't waste energy. Don't even consider stopping. Remove it as a concept. Replace 'stop' with 'keep going'. Steady rhythm. Nothing hasty. The good zone to be in. The good place.

What Freya loved about the path round the fields was that a full circuit got her up to about ten K on the nose, give or take a tenth or so. She wasn't particularly bothered about getting a good time in, so long as she got the distance behind her. The fitness tracker – her mother's last Christmas gift to her – told her that her resting pulse rate was excellent, putting her in the same zone as professional athletes, but for Freya it was less about streams of figures and sellable personal data, and more about the steady routine – The Plod, was her term for it – and the glow of endorphins after she finished. It was habit-forming, she knew.

The farmer's path was perhaps her favourite route of the three she went on regularly, although they all had merits and drawbacks. The canal path was a good all-rounder, and didn't tend to pool puddles or have too much mud – a long, straight path, and some ducks to look at. But there was heavy traffic in its narrow confines, too many fellow runners, cyclists, dog walkers or just people out stretching their legs. As in many other things, Freya was an intensely private person, particularly when it came to running. She'd never encountered anyone on the canal path who was up to no good, and there'd only been one or two catcalls from troglodyte males on the other side of the water; but too many people simply didn't suit Freya.

The route around the back of the houses and up and down the ginnels and through the parkland was mostly private, but also enclosed and constricted, with a sense of danger that she could never quite shake. There had been no Minotaur lurking in that labyrinth, but there was always the sense that there might be one. The regularity of the fences and the general good condition of the houses was a plus, but this was at the expense of open ground and a bigger sky, two things that she had come to value on her runs.

That's why the farmer's field was her favourite. She'd

discovered it on a website for runners, although she very rarely saw them on the land. The farmer was relaxed about open access to the paths, although Freya sometimes despaired at the empty water bottles, discarded dog bags and other detritus that she came across. It ran along the fringes of a variety of crops – barley, wheat, even rhubarb in its Triffid-like stalks, grown taller than Freya in the warm months before they were cropped – and if the weather had been dry for a few days, it was a delight. It curved up towards some woodland, which provided a pleasing contrast to the flat open plane, and her ankles and knees always thanked her rejection of concrete in favour of less rigid terrain. This latter quality ensured that it could get boggy, even treacherous in patches if the grips on her trainers had worn smooth. She had come home in some appalling states, a fine workout for her washing machine, but today promised a drier time of it.

Push through. Push on.

She sometimes used music, although just as often she disappeared into her imagination. As she skirted the edge of the woods, heading towards the stony path that took her through the treeline, she made sure the player was off. Though she never felt any sense of threat in the woods, it was still a lonely place, and Freya knew it paid to be wary.

On. Step up the incline; take the strain. Tight at the calves. Head down. Grit teeth. Step up and push through.

Freya was sweating freely as the trees closed in. Occasionally she had to beware the odd patch of nettles or leap over the groping crimson tentacles of bramble bushes, and dog mess was a constant danger – an unfortunate side effect of having a farm so close to a built-up area – all a help, all keeping her supple and fit, and largely calm.

That was the day that she saw the arrows. They had been carved in the bark of an ash tree not yet blighted with the dieback she'd noticed in other wooded areas. At first the intrusion on the texture of the trees had annoyed her – regularity in a place where it was unnatural. An arrow, pointing to right, leaving an oozing raw patch bleeding sap, like fresh skin after a plaster is ripped off. The arrow was telling Freya to follow her usual path, and she only felt a sense of unease, rather than dread. It did not occur to her that this patrin was meant for her, until she trudged past it, and noticed that a name had been carved underneath the arrow.

FREYA.

She stopped, and ripped the earbuds from her ears. A scan of the trees, a kaleidoscope of browns and greens as she spun around. No one. Not that she could see, anyway.

She carried on, muscles aching from the sudden braking. Her heart rate had picked up, and there was no need to check her fitness tracker to be sure of that.

A second arrow urged her to change direction, down a more overgrown path that she had followed once, and not enjoyed. It, too had 'FREYA' carved underneath, in thick capital letters.

'Don't be an idiot,' she whispered to herself. But the trees thinned out into birches and pines, nothing that someone could easily hide behind. Even if they lay in the grass or the bushes, there were no thickets close to the path, weed-choked and generally overgrown as it was. After ducking past some overhanging branches, she reached a huge old oak, its bough twisted like a lightning bolt, with an immense bole at its centre.

Above this bole, there was another arrow. This one was pointing downwards. Again, her name was attached underneath.

Something white was inside the bole.

Now, the oak was big enough for someone to hide behind, for sure. Freya took her time, giving it a wide berth, feet crunching through a carpet of detritus and pine needles, circling the immense tree. No one hid behind it. No one hid in it, either – she thought, for one horrible moment, that someone might be perched on a branch, squeezed in among the natural forks and crossbeams like a leopard, preparing to pounce. But she was alone here, surely.

She approached the bole. There was an envelope, sealed up in a plastic zip-lock bag. Even through the clear plastic, she could make out her name, inked in the same blocky lettering on the front of the envelope.

Freya took it out by her fingertips, dropping it to the forest floor. She crouched, darting quick glances towards the trees, sweat cooling on her brow, as she unlocked the bag and brought out the envelope.

It was unsealed, the protective paper still stuck to the gummed edge. Inside was a piece of paper with a printed-out message on it at the top, in black ink.

It read: On the middle fork, you go past the hanging oak. Then you prove your mettle.

She heard footsteps on the trail behind her. Freya threw the letter into the zip-lock bag, stuffed it into the pocket of her training top, and began to run, darting through the trees towards the main path.

There was a man behind her – dressed in dark clothes, and running fast. Panic flooded through her, her feet hitting the trail hard, the trees a blur, before the man shouted:

'Hey, Freya – wait!'

12

The worst thing was, she didn't run far. She got away from the tree and the oozing arrows, but her path took her into a thicket. She turned and faced the man who ran after her.

He slipped through the trees, nightmarishly sinuous, shoulders fluid as they turned this way and that to admit him. Where Freya would probably have tripped over, or had her face striped by branches. He had a thin face with a pointy chin, and long dark hair shot through with grey that made him look like a busker who had weathered well, or a rock star who had weathered badly. He was tall, dressed in black except for a reflective neon bib, and athletic. He had his training bottoms tucked into thoroughbred white cotton sports socks.

Freya shrank away in terror. 'What do you want... what do you want with me?'

He stopped and raised a hand. He was out of breath and sweating, and looked as if he had been running as long as Freya had. 'I can explain,' he said, taking deep breaths. 'I'm Detective Inspector Connor Tamm. I'm a police officer. I'm actually off-duty... This is awkward. Wait.'

The man reached into a pocket and brought out some ID.

He held it out to Freya, as a tourist might hold out a biscuit to a baboon on holiday. Freya made no motion to take the card, but from that distance she could see that the name and the face matched up on the ID.

'I've never seen a warrant card before – that could have come out of a Christmas cracker. What do you want from me?'

'I couldn't get a hold of you, and there's no number for you listed on any database. I spoke to a neighbour who told me you ran – the lady who lives across the hall. She said that on Tuesdays, you head over to the farmer's fields.'

'So you followed me? What for?'

'It isn't like that…' Then he sighed, and placed his hands on his back. 'OK. It is like that. I just wanted to check in and say hello. It has been brought to my attention that you published a newspaper article on your… relationship with Gareth Solomon.'

'He's my father. You don't need to skate around it.' Freya had still to calm down. The fear had not subsided. The man made a show of staying back and keeping his hands empty, but Freya felt boxed in among the trees. She could force herself through the thicket, but he would surely catch up with her before she did so.

'I just wanted to remind you that there is an appeal ongoing in his case. You can't prejudice a judge in the Supreme Court, but I want you to be wary, going forward. I wanted to speak to you when I was in plain clothes, and not like this… But this isn't a formal interview, or anything.'

'Social call, is it? You just about scared me out of my mind!'

'I'm sorry.' Tamm looked as if this hadn't occurred to him. 'I apologise. I don't have the time in working hours to wait to contact someone – I just wanted to catch up with you informally. And, incidentally, to find a new running route. This is a gem, isn't it?'

'It's great – but you didn't go to this effort to talk about running, did you? What is it you want?'

'We'd appreciate it if you pass on anything you can find out from your father about the Woodcutter case. Whether he's guilty of killing June Caton-Bell or not, we believe he was guilty of the other murders, an attempted murder and one or two other missing persons cases. Any detail you find that either exonerates him or proves his guilt – you have to turn it over to us. Now I know you're a sensible, clever lass, and you wouldn't get any ideas about Gareth Solomon after meeting the man twice…'

'What ideas would those be?'

'Any ideas at all. If you find out anything, let me know. Also, please be careful if you're putting your face out in the open – there are a lot of bad actors out there.'

'Yeah. Most of them play policemen at some point.'

He had the grace to laugh. 'I'll leave a card, Freya. You don't have to come over and get it… Look, I'll stick it here.' Tamm dropped a white business card down in between the bark and the spiky branches of a young conifer, then backed away. 'We should talk soon. Anything you can turn out on the Woodcutter is a help. I'll let you get on with your run, and I'm sorry if I startled you.'

Freya said nothing, waiting until the dark figure had returned to the path before running back the way it came. Freya scooped up the business card, then headed in the other direction, travelling along the stony path as fast as she could until she was clear of the trees.

13

Hello…

Yes, hello. I'm talking to you. Blimey, you look confused, love. Have you been crying?

Ah – you are crying. All right. That's OK. Just, take your time… There's no rush. Nice deep breaths…

Who's that, now? Who are you calling for? No, that's not me. Dunno who that is. Sounds like a nice person. Sounds like you miss them.

Your mum? Oh God. Don't call for your mum. For goodness' sake. That's pathetic. Stop it or I'll end you right now. You got it? I'm going to open the door and… Look, I'll fucking split you down the middle. Got it? That's what I'll do. Stop the snivelling. I hate that more than anything. Stop the… That's better. OK. Just sit up a minute. Yes, I can see you. Hello! Imagine me waving. I'm waving at you. That's it. Well done. Yeah. You look a bit weird in night vision. But to be honest it's not a brilliant look for anyone.

Hear that sound? That scratchy sound? That's me, grinding the side of my axe against the paintwork. Don't worry about the paintwork; it's only an old banger. This heap of shit's going to end up the size of a hamburger before long. Heh! Want to hear it again?

That's right. I said 'axe'.

Yeah. Take a moment, won't you? Let it sink in. It's a lot. You know, I had someone one time, when I got a hold of them and put them under, they didn't survive. Big guy. Had a kind of rugby look to him. Turned out he had asthma or something. No one ever found out about him. One of many little projects. I was really upset, in fact. Anyhow. You lasted longer than him, you've got that going for you. You've come through that. You're ahead of the game. Look sharp, look lively!

You had a very interesting skirt on, so I took the liberty of taking it off you while you were sleeping. Don't worry, it isn't as weird as it sounds. It's for your benefit. You see, I know you're a runner. I've been watching you. Tonight was my big chance. And you can't run with a skirt like that on. Nice floral number. Very boho. Except you'd be like a fucking Dalek, if you have to run in it. You'll trip. And if you trip and fall, well…

Scritch, scratch. I like that sound. It sets some people's teeth on edge. Not mine.

Right, here's the deal. I'll open the door, I'll cut the cable ties, and I'll give you a chance to escape. When the door's open, take a moment to familiarise yourself with your surroundings. There's not much to it. It's some shithole that got demolished and left to the rats and the weeds. There's no fucker here. Trees and stuff in the background. Piles of crappy old industrial units. We are parked inside what I believe was once a tyres and exhausts place. Some interesting bits and pieces lying around. If you were especially brave, you can find one and use it as a weapon. Someone did that once, you know. Found a bit of scaffolding. Used it as a quarterstaff.

I was genuinely flummoxed – I couldn't get near that bitch for a while. I was going to award her the match, and scarper. Brave lass. She still fucking died, screaming. Are you that brave? I think I can see an old wrench lying there. It could just be a dead squirrel or something. Everything tends to brown – wrenches. Dead squirrels. Blood. Your blood, in fact.

You can scream your head off, if you like. We are totally alone. There's no one to help you.

Right, I'm going to give you a countdown. I'll let you listen to the birdies – all sorts, around here. Such a peaceful sound, isn't it? The wind rustling the leaves and branches. Birdies tweeting outside. This might be your last chance to hear them. Sit up, and listen. Just listen. Take it all in.

Only joking. Here I come!

14

Glenn Allander was a fair man, with a floppy fringe drumming its fingers above a high, clear brow and outsized glasses. He was a little under average height, but was striking-looking, quite fit. There wasn't much fat on his face but there was still a cute chunkiness in it, thanks to his high cheekbones and a square jaw. Those were cheeks you might pinch. He had a rounded chin and a full mouth, and might still look boyish when he reached his forties. There could be a Kal-El hiding there, not too far from the surface.

Freya cycled past him twice, and he barely noticed as he walked down the street, seemingly engrossed in whatever he was listening to on his earbuds. The wiring trailed from an inside coat pocket, and he seemed in a hurry, constantly looking over his shoulder.

She locked up her bike at some railings near the coffee shop. The place wasn't part of a big chain, and judging by the stacked stools on some of the tables, it wasn't going to be open too much longer. Freya kept her helmet and shades on as she watched him take a seat, his back to the wall. He ordered a bottle of water and sipped at it, then tapped at his phone.

Her own phone buzzed soon after. 'In position,' read the text message.

Definitely him, then. That was good. No one following him, like a photographer; that was better.

She took off her helmet and kept it under her arms, and ordered a coffee.

He looked up, and peered at her for a second or two, before going back to his phone.

He frowned when she approached, cutting through a patch of fading sunlight cast across the floor. 'Uh… Freya?'

She smiled. 'Yes, Freya Bain. You must be Glenn?'

He seemed surprised as he stood up to greet her, shaking hands tentatively. 'Gads, you're taller than I thought. Changed your hair, too.'

'You could say I'm in disguise.'

'Tabloids been after you?'

She nodded. 'Price I paid for going public. I've turned into news. It's… weird.'

Glenn Allander sat down, still keeping his back to the wall. 'Did you ride a bike here?'

Freya pinched some of her Day-Glo yellow fitness gear. 'Course. This isn't my usual night-out gear.'

'No, it's just that… I could've sworn you cycled past me.'

'Probably did.'

'I mean, more than once.' He drummed his fingers. 'Anyone would think you were stalking me.'

'Well, one good turn deserves another.'

'I wouldn't have connected you with… well, you. God, you look so different.'

'Funny what a change of hairstyle can do for a girl. That, plus different eyeshadow.'

'You've got his eyes, all the same. Your dad's eyes.'

'They all say that. So… sorry for the cloak and dagger. But I guess you started it.'

'Quite. It was a bit of a breakthrough for me, I have to say. There's always been doubt about your father's conviction. I've always thought so, anyway.' He took a swallow of his water. Steady hand, Freya noticed.

'You don't look too much older than me. What are you, about twenty-eight?'

'Yeah. In a couple of months.'

'But your Red Ink thing… that's been going for years. I mean, you'd have been at school when you started it.'

'That's right.' He blinked, once.

'It's kind of detailed… crime scene photos, and whatnot. Didn't you get sued?'

'Not at all. A takedown notice. Hardly the same thing. I complied.'

Freya paused. She felt supremely awkward, as if the balance of the exchange had tipped in his favour. Certainly he was a cool customer, clipped and controlled. 'Now, about this police officer. I hadn't heard much about it from the case.'

'The PC? Who had an affair with your dad? Yeah that's a strange one. According to some notes on the case and one or two police officers we spoke to, your father was in a relationship with Carol Ramirez. No one knows quite how it started, how they got together, but they had a relationship when he was passing through. There's some talk that he was in a pub one night when a fight broke out, she attended the scene, and he managed to chat her up there and then, when she was dealing with it. There is a long-standing rumour that on the night June Caton-Bell was killed, he was with her the whole night. That she's his alibi. That's the night that the eyewitness supposedly saw him getting into and out of the van, apparently after he chopped Caton-Bell up.

'But Carol Ramirez never turned up since, in the inquiry, never gave evidence in the trial, and there was some kind of legal reason that they didn't mention her in his defence. It's never been properly explained, but there's something weird about it. Anyway… it turns out that the guy in charge of the Woodcutter inquiry knew about it, and got her to make some kind of statement, denying she had anything to do with him, that he was a fantasist. She was supposedly on duty that night, in another part of town. It totally flies in the face of the rumours.'

'Slow down a minute,' Freya said. 'You're saying that my father could have proved he was with a woman… a *policewoman*, in fact… on the night June Caton-Bell was killed? And somehow that was never revealed during his trial? And it's never come to light, until now?'

'That's what I understand.'

'So, she could clear him?'

'That's the thinking. I reckon that's the key part of the appeal going through the courts at the moment.'

'How did you find out all this?'

'Same way any news portal does. I got a tip. I saw a redacted document. It was sent to me, anonymously.'

'You didn't say anything about that in the article I read about Carol Ramirez.'

'I have to protect my source.' Glenn drained the last of his bottle, then screwed on the top. 'It's most likely a serving copper.'

'Most likely Carol Ramirez, you mean?'

'Not out of the question.' A flicker of a smile, as he brushed his fringe away from his eyes. 'Anyway. That coffee smells good. I don't usually bother with coffee, this close to bedtime. I'm tempted, though. Can I get you something else?'

'How about something stronger?'

'Oh, hell yeah.' He grinned. His face was transformed. 'Is it still drink driving if you're in charge of a bike, can I ask?'

'No idea. Shall we find out?'

The place called itself *Byzantium* and had taken a creditable stab at ancient Turkish-themed décor. It was a restaurant, but rowdy with it, with a separate bar section that catered for its own clientele.

Freya almost wished they'd stayed in the coffee shop. The music was tolerable, but only just. The clientele were mostly office workers, all of them far more stylish than either Glenn or Freya. Her highlighter-pen Lycra and her pinned-back blonde hair got one or two dirty looks, which she had giggled at.

Freya had to raise her voice to be heard properly. The hubbub robbed Glenn of his confidence, but it had only taken a couple of pints to replace it in his pockets.

She snapped off the edge of a slice of pizza and nodded towards a painted skyline that showed minarets against a purpling sky. 'Don't think Istanbul's skyline and boozing quite goes together, I dunno about you.'

'This place is a mess, and it's too loud – but I like the booths. Private, you know?' He sipped his pint; she noticed that he'd hardly touched his food; nor had he removed his jacket, although it was hot in there. 'I've got a local we could go to. Proper fish and chips. Pies with a crust you need a chisel to get through. Old men and dark beer. Awful toilets.'

'Maybe next time.' She smiled, not unkindly. 'Let's go back to the theory. Tell me how my dad didn't do it.'

'Well... On the Caton-Bell case, the one he was convicted for, there's reasonable doubt. There is some evidence to suggest he is circumstantially tied to the places where the other victims disappeared from, though. Not enough to bring charges. He was in transit at the time, working as a courier.'

'Caton-Bell, though. What's the theory?'

'Well. She was out running, and someone snatched her off an A-road. Quiet place; no traffic. It was a baffling case, and it was quickly linked to the others. Except this time, someone called the cops to talk about a man seen getting into a black van near thc woods where her body was discovered. She picked out your father in the ID line-up, then testified that it was him in court.'

'What reason do you have to doubt her?'

'Well...' Glenn sipped at his pint like a bird pecking at a pint of milk on a doorstep. 'She came into some money not long after all this.'

'What, you mean... Someone bribed her? To fit my dad up?'

'All I'm saying is, she came into some money. And she bought a touring caravan, which she wrote off about six weeks later. She didn't win the lottery, she didn't get a bonus at work, and it arrived in the form of cash. When she went to the dealership, she handed over used notes.'

'How do you know this stuff?'

'I'm not bad at investigations.' Glenn said this, matter-of-fact, without a trace of defensiveness or bluster. 'And as I say, I pick up tips all the time.'

'What are you? You work in the police, or the law, or… what?'

He actually blushed. 'I work in data. Figures, statistics, research. Numbers, you know.'

'Wow. Is it totally awful?'

'Unbelievably bad,' he said, without hesitation. 'Put it this way – I look into old murders and that's *leisure*.'

After she'd stopped laughing, Freya asked: 'You reckon she fitted him up, on someone else's behalf?'

'I'll admit it's a possibility. If I was your father, it's something I'd want to look into.'

'Does he know about this?'

'He should.'

'When did this come out? The stuff about the witness?'

'Her name's Grace Parminter. She's still alive. Lives alone in a cottage. Crazy lady, so they say. Lots of cats. Though that doesn't mean anything. Partial to the odd cat, myself.'

'I bet you are.' She finished another piece of pizza, then reached for his. 'Sorry, I'm in training. You're not going to eat that, are you?'

'Nah. I had a big lunch. Eyes bigger than my belly.'

Freya shrugged, and scooped up a slice. 'Don't be afraid of carbs. They have power, if used wisely.'

Glenn said nothing, taking a small sip at his pint. While she ate, he glanced over towards a bar, where golden-skinned young women were shrieking with laughter as they all depth-charged shots. A mirrored tile warped reality over his shoulder. In this woozy portal, Freya saw her eyes dance as she ate and drank. *Steady*, she thought. *Nothing crazy, here*.

She could feel the drink running away with her blood, and part of her reason. Freya wasn't much of a drinker, but she knew the treachery of lowered inhibitions. At times when she was younger she'd gotten too drunk, too quickly. It had cost her friends, or earned her disdain from competitors. She'd learned the hard way. She'd limit herself to one or two, tops.

'So you reckon that's going to emerge during his appeal?'

'I couldn't possibly say.'

'Who did you talk to? Was it my dad's lawyer? Levison? She seems a bit of a loose cannon.'

'Persistent, aren't you?' Glenn grinned. She liked that grin. He had nice, white, even teeth. She doubted his story about drinking too much coffee at work. 'I'm not going to tell you. Best not to ask.'

'If we're going to work together, then you have to tell me some stuff.'

'Who said we're going to work together?'

'I'm saying it, now. I want to clear my dad. If you give me what you know, he'll be out of jail before we know it.'

'Interesting offer.'

'He might even come and talk to you. You could interview him. An exclusive. How about that?'

'How well do you know him? From what I read, you've only met him the once. Like – in your entire life. You don't know him at all.'

'That's true, but I have met him. Twice. Which puts me ahead of you. And, hey, key point – I'm his daughter.'

'You can prove that? Sorry, I mean no offence, it's just… you've got dark eyes. What I can see of them. They look like his eyes. That's not proof, though.'

'You'll have to see, won't you? It's all in hand. That could be another exclusive for you.'

'Interesting. I'll bear it in mind. And get an answer to you – when we're sober.'

'You're all business.' Freya drained her pint. 'I like that, believe it or not.'

'I'm glad. You'll appreciate what I say next, then. I'm going to be up-front.'

She laughed, much too loud. 'Now I'm officially goddamned intrigued!'

Glenn placed both hands on the table in front of him, as if to steady himself. 'I think your father has an excellent case, if he appeals his conviction. There is reasonable doubt that he was fitted up in the Caton-Bell case, probably by the police in charge. They've got previous for it. And reasonable doubt is enough to get him out of jail. But in terms of the Woodcutter case, and the other missing people… I have every suspicion that he snatched them in the same way, and there's every chance he was the person who killed them.'

'I know that,' she said, casually. 'All a matter of legal terminology and technical detail though, isn't it? I mean… No bodies. No proof. No witnesses. Just a bunch of dates and coincidences in terms of his courier job. That goes for him and thousands of other long-distance drivers. How many times a week do truckers go up and down the major motorways?'

'I get all that,' Glenn conceded. 'To be clear, I don't have a firm opinion one way or the other. I go by the facts, and

I raise questions where they need asking. When things don't make sense, I say so. In the Caton-Bell case, there are inconsistencies that have never been explained. That makes me doubtful. But only in terms of the conviction. I don't have much doubt that he's a killer.'

'Very forensic. I noticed that about your Red Ink site. You're big into the science of it. That ties in with the data and statistics, I guess.'

He shrugged. 'I suppose. It's not all raw science, though. Tips can help. I have put away a couple of people. You know that, right?'

Freya lifted her glass; he clinked it with his own, reluctantly. 'Oh, I know it. You got the guy who shot that shopkeeper. Mentioned in dispatches by the police, and all sorts. Though secretly I bet they hate you. You made them look a bit daft.'

'Oh, they hate me, all right.' He grinned again. 'Don't doubt it.'

'What's your thing, then?'

'My… thing?'

'Yeah. What is it that you're into? I would have said, you have an unhealthy fascination with murder. So does everybody. It's not that unusual. But they don't start some white knight website because of it. What's the deal? Why do you do it? You must have built this website when you were at school. And the detail is… unbelievable. *Forensic* is the word. Chemistry, the pure science of it, the pathologists' reports… It's so dense it seems like a medical textbook, rather than a website for murder junkies. So, what is it? What's the juice?'

'The juice, as you put it, is to do with unsolved crimes.

I don't like people getting away with murder. I don't like people suffering, knowing that guy who killed their loved one is still out there. And above all, I don't like innocent people being blamed for things they didn't do. I want the baddies caught. So that's my thing. Seeing as you asked.' Glenn finished his pint and folded his arms.

Finally. A reaction.

'Want to get out of here?' she asked.

'What, again?' He sighed. 'Look, I'm tired, I've had a long week at work…'

'I'm sorry.' She coloured. 'I'll be honest, it's a long time since I had a night out.'

'Well, this is just, you know. A couple of pints after work. No big deal.'

'Totally,' she said, much too quickly. 'No big deal at all. You OK with doing it again? Go over some notes, or whatever?'

She could have died at his expression, right then. Utter incredulity. Then she noticed he had begun to blush, too. 'Sure. We can get back next week. That's a date. I mean, we'll make a date for it. In our diaries, thing. Um.'

'You're right, definitely. Let's swap numbers. I'll choose the next place, if you don't mind. And – it's your round.'

'You sure about that?' He grinned, slyly.

Freya drained her glass. 'There's one other thing to say. It might sound mad…'

'Go on,' he said, cautiously, his drink paused on its way up to his mouth.

'Well. I had this message. Anonymous. I won't say exactly how I got it, but… I've had some kind of, what you'd call, I guess…' She exhaled. 'A tip.'

'A tip? About your dad?'

'I don't know. Look – we should probably wrap this up. This is going to my head. One pint. Jesus.'

'You've had three. Listen, you said you'd had a tip?' His fingers were a blur on his phone. He was making a note. 'When did you get it?'

She felt a sense of horror, as if a trapdoor fell somewhere in her guts. *Said too much. Shouldn't have said that. After one pint! With one boy!*

'Look, I said I have to go. It's fine. We'll talk later.'

'Well, can we share a cab? Where do you stay?'

'It's fine, I've got a bike. I don't think I'm drunk enough to get stopped by the police. Shit… am I?'

'I'll call you tomorrow,' he said. 'That be OK?'

'Sure. Any time.'

15

A hangover. Despite not having so much to drink. Possibly it was just shame. Shame at the ebullience. At being out and about. At saying intensely, unbearably stupid things. She'd said too much. Her baseline was cringe. That was her starter for 10. Had she really said anything bad? She didn't think so. God, she hadn't even had too much to drink.

No. Wait. She'd told him…

Freya was staring at her phone, sitting on the edge of her bed, thinking about a text to compose, when he rang, right there, out of the blue.

'Everything OK?' was the only thing she could think to say.

'Well… Yeah. Suppose. I meant to say – I'd been thinking. About the tip you got. Anything more you can tell me? It might be important. I could help.'

He could help. That was the thing. Freya did need an ally. That ally wasn't Mick Harvie; Freya felt like he'd be a better fit. 'Sure. It was a message. In the woods. I know that sounds…'

'In the woods?' he spluttered. 'What was it, the Blair Witch?'

'It sounds silly, but believe it – there was a message left for me, on my running route, through the woods, and it told me: *On the middle fork, you go past the hanging oak. Then you prove your mettle.*' Freya stared through the net curtains onto the busy street below the flat. 'There are a couple of vague hits on the internet, but I thought we could talk it through, later. I suppose we got sidetracked.'

Glenn sighed. 'This is all difficult to believe, I have to say. Some random note, left for you in the woods?'

'It wasn't random. Sounds specific, wouldn't you say? I think someone's been stalking me.'

'And your stalker left you some sort of Simon Says puzzle?' He sighed.

'You can believe it or not, but that's what happened. It can't be a coincidence after I appeared in the press. There was another thing…' She told him about DI Tamm.

His reaction was not unexpected. 'What! And some copper happened to appear… I mean, what am I expected to think about this? You're not even sure he was a copper?'

'DI Connor Tamm – I looked him up. He's attached to loads of press releases. Worked on murder cases, gangland stuff. It's definitely him.'

'Christ, that is peculiar. Basically stalking you? Why wouldn't he keep you under surveillance?'

'He said the police are skint.'

'That, I buy,' he said, in a less febrile tone. 'You reckon he suspects something?'

'No idea,' Freya said, picturing the police officer with the neon bib. 'They all think they're Columbo. Which is fine, unless they act like it. He was a bit of an enigma.'

'So, the note… what are you saying? This was the actual

Woodcutter, come to give you a clue? Why would he do that?'

'I don't know what was going on, or who did it. I'm just telling you what happened. It could be some twisted arsehole. It could have been the Woodcutter. For all I know, it could have been you.'

'Nice.'

'I'm sorry.' Freya flushed with shame. 'I didn't mean that. I'm a bit stressed.'

'It's fine. Understandable. OK. We'll talk about it. What exactly did the note say, again?'

'He said, "On the middle fork, you go past the hanging oak. Then you prove your mettle."' It almost felt embarrassing, said aloud, like a magic spell for a child.

'Someone left you a bloody crossword puzzle? Two down, three letters, does the splits? Forgive my cynicism.'

'Take it or leave it. Give me a call when you stop wasting my time. Forgive my impatience.' She stabbed the disconnect button.

Freya watched buses seem to kiss each other as they stopped, seemingly nose to nose, at opposite ends of the road. At this time of day, the people on board looked particularly grim. Older folk, students, mothers with clambering children. She was going to tear the net curtains down, soon. She'd already rearranged the furniture in the front room, and was going to have the carpet replaced. Soon it would feel like it was hers.

The phone rang. It was Glenn.

'Look, I'm...' He took a breath, held it, then said: 'Sorry.'

'You're fine. No big deal.'

'Right. Listen, I've been thinking… you said you had some internet hits for a place?'

'Yeah, one or two places in the UK.'

'When I made the crossword puzzle joke, it got me to thinking. If he was giving you some kind of cryptic clue to follow, then it wouldn't give you lots of options to waste your time on. It could be Timbuktu, for all you know, if it was something vague, possibly global. You're probably quite close with a basic internet search. It's promising. I'll get on it, then get back to you.'

Neither of them had a car. On Glenn's day off, a couple of days later, they took a train then a Toytown bus service over undulating country roads. Freya felt she was in a children's stop-motion animation as the bus heaved and wheezed up and down narrow roads.

They were the only passengers for much of the journey. Watching the farmland on either side, with barely a house to be seen, the crops still low in the early springtime, Freya grew uncomfortable.

Glenn had put on a podcast; seeing Freya's uncomfortable expression, he pulled out his earbuds. 'What's up?'

'I don't like this. It could be a complete wild goose chase.'

'Could be. But at least we're checking it out.'

'I'm thinking that calling the cops was probably the best idea. They could have done something. Forensics. Fingerprints. Tweezers. That sort of thing.'

'I did say you should call the police.'

'Yeah, but not very convincingly.'

Glenn shrugged. 'It's what I would have done. Probably.'

Freya nudged him, and smiled. 'You're not the world's best liar.'

'What do you mean?'

'I mean, you're obviously as into this as I am.'

'If you get a lead, you follow it through.' He shrugged, and looked away. 'Best to check it out. This was the best hit we got.'

'I think you were reaching. Just a little bit.'

'I wasn't reaching at all. It was a reasonable deduction, based on what you told me. This was our best bet.'

'So, you basically typed "Middle Fork" and "Hanging Oak" into a search engine, and you got this place?'

'It was a tiny bit more involved, than that. I worked it back the other way. I searched for "Hanging Oak", first. There's even a pub called *The Hanging Oak*, can you believe that? "Families welcome – two for one on Sunday lunch at *The Hanging Oak*". I then got a little bit sidetracked, looking for pubs with dodgy names. *The Spurting Stump*, *The Cold Embrace of the Grave*, that sort of thing.' When Freya didn't laugh, he continued: 'I crossed that off the list, first. Not much to link that with anything called the Middle Fork. So I indexed all the places that listed "the Hanging Oak". There were quite a few of these, but that's when I put it together. Looking at them with just the term "fork" took me to a place called Devil's Fork Road. This is close to an actual hanging oak. In fact… We're coming up to it… Christ, I think this is it.' Suddenly he got to his feet, ringing the bell and pulling his backpack off the overhead rack.

They were almost immediately beset by tiny flies as they got off at a bus stop fashioned out of drystone, a bunker set before a wall, complete with a mossy slate bench. Freya supposed this was meant to look organic, but it just came off as creepy. A troll lives there, she thought.

Glenn heaved the rucksack over his shoulder, grimacing at the weight. It was one of those Nordic trekker numbers, too big and too long for an average back, perhaps better suited to a polar bear's. Inside it, metallic things grated and clanked. 'Now we've got a bit of a walk.' He indicated the road stretching up ahead, as the bus crept out of sight around a corner.

Freya glanced over her shoulder at the empty road. 'There's no pavements. And the road seems narrow. And we can't see what's coming when it goes around a bend. We could get squished, here.'

'Exciting, isn't it?'

Any excitement either of them felt was gone after an hour. The day was overcast but it had an unpleasant, muggy heat, as if the late morning was giving serious consideration to a storm. They had to look lively over a course of about three miles, stepping to the other side of the road as a bus came in the opposite direction.

'Here's a maths question,' Freya said. 'Two trucks coming in opposite directions. In the exact point that they pass each other, we'll be in their way. My question is, how fast do you think you could climb that wall?'

'Fast enough, if it came to it,' Glenn said. She doubted it, though. She noticed he was sweating freely. She'd offered to take the backpack off him, but he'd scowled at her in that almost cute, petulant way of his at the suggestion. He wasn't quite so fit as he looked, she thought, but at least he was a gentleman.

Glenn palmed sweat off his brow, then squinted at the

curving road up ahead. 'Right – I think there's a way in... Just up here. Oh, hello.'

'What?'

'There's a lay-by. It's not obvious on the online maps... It wasn't on the OS, either.'

'I thought it was a ditch.'

'You could definitely park something there.'

'Why would you want to?'

Glenn didn't reply. He didn't have to.

'That'll be our way in, then,' she said.

It might have been a turnstile of some kind; there was a gate, but its bars were rusted into twisted ruin. A giant might have twisted these, for fun. The hinge just about worked; it gouged out a fresh furrow in the dank turf.

'Nancy Drew says, no one's come through here in a good while,' Freya said, indicating the freshly scarred turf.

Glenn nodded. 'This all kind of ties in.'

'You going to talk in riddles all day, or are you going to explain yourself?'

He huffed and straightened the backpack on his shoulders, as they faced an open, fallow field, becoming slightly overgrown with the burgeoning spring. There was not a living creature to be seen aside from the flies. 'Well,' Glenn said, 'this ties in with a long-standing theory about the Woodcutter. The reason I haven't explained all this is because, well, I kind of assumed you would have studied all this.'

Freya held her tongue.

He continued: 'So, stop me if you've heard any of this before. The theory is that, given what happened to June Caton-Bell, the Woodcutter kidnapped people out on their own, alone. Men, women – they were all quite strong. Runners. Ex-military, a guy who could handle himself. He incapacitated them, somehow. The post-mortem on Caton-Bell's remains showed she hadn't been drugged, but might have been knocked out. Blow to the head, maybe. So the thinking is that the Woodcutter woke his victims up, and set them free. He gave them a head start. And then he chased them.

'That was the juice. He wanted to run them down. Then, when he caught up with them… You know the rest.'

'Is it possible the Woodcutter took one of them out here?'

Glenn indicated the desolate plain before them. 'What do you reckon?'

'I reckon maybe.'

They carried on in silence, before their path was ended by a drystone wall. There was a stile set into the crags and outcroppings, basically a set of iron slabs protruding from the rock. None of this looked particularly safe; it creaked when Freya placed her foot on the first rung, and she expected it to crumble as if made of gingerbread. But they clambered over quickly enough. This crossed into even wilder meadowland. Dandelions poked their head out of the grasses, but this was no wildflower-strewn arboreal idyll; the place looked sick, neglected.

'Swampy in here,' Glenn said, glancing at his boots after one good big squelch.

'I think there's a trail of some kind up there.'

'Yeah. And I think what we're looking for is right over there, in the other field.'

He gestured, but Freya had to squint to make it out. 'The Hanging Oak?'

Glenn nodded, somewhat smugly. 'Yeah. That's the one, right there.'

'It's got character, that's for sure.' There was something particularly forbidding about the stunted shape in the distance, a black, twisted knot on the horizon. It was as if it had noticed them. It looked poised to break into a run, Freya thought.

'My thinking is that the Woodcutter might have taken one of his victims out here,' Glenn said. 'Looking at the wider map, this was either Coleen Arden, or Max Dilworth. Draw a circle around the abduction sites, and plot the points, then those are two closest locations to here.'

'If that's true, then this person who got in touch with me… is the actual Woodcutter?'

'It's a possibility,' Glenn said, after some consideration.

The horror of it dawned on her. She fed off his unease. 'I mean, what does he want with me? And how does he know where I live? Where I run?'

'You can't be sure of that.'

'Oh come on – he knew where I run, for definite. The message was left for me. So was the puzzle.' She swallowed. It was beginning to dawn on her. Out there, just outside Freya's periphery, a hunter was sizing her up, making assessments, taking notes. And playing games. 'What does he want?'

'I wouldn't leap to conclusions,' Glenn said. 'There's lots of possibilities, here. If it is the Woodcutter, he's taking a hell of a risk.'

'Who else could it be?'

'Maybe your dad's trying to get messages to you. Point

you in the way of the bodies. Maybe he thinks it's helping him get out of jail.'

'That would make no sense at all. Who'd be doing it?'

'He's not short of admirers. Maybe even his lawyer. Make it look like the real Woodcutter's out there.'

'That doesn't make me feel safe, either. Either it's the Woodcutter or someone who writes letters to him. God, this is a mess.' She had a sudden fantasy, vivid as moonlight breaching the clouds; her being startled awake, and a dark figure standing at the end of her bed. *I'll never sleep again.*

Glenn's eyes seemed feverish behind his glasses, and he chewed his lips. He was enmeshed in his own world, his own fantasies, for a moment. 'Well, a clue's a clue. Whoever gave us it, we can work with it. For my money, there's a good chance it's the real Woodcutter. Or at least, the guy who killed Coleen Arden and Max Dilworth.'

'So you're saying that my dad could be innocent? He might be telling the truth?'

'I'm just investigating a tip from you, based on a weird encounter. This could be nothing. My mind is filling in a lot of blanks, here. That's one theory. But I'll believe nothing until I see it. We've got to keep our eyes peeled, focus...'

'Hey, we've got company.' Freya nodded towards something ambling towards them over the lip of a hill. It was a dun-coloured cow. Its shoulders moved in a distinctly un-bovine manner, its massive shoulder muscles folding in on each other as it approached. 'Nice to see some signs of life.'

Glenn stopped. 'Signs. We passed a sign, didn't we?'

'Not sure I remember that.'

There was a beat or two.

'I think there was a sign, all snarled up in the bushes, near that stile. I didn't pay too much attention to it. Was there some yellow in that sign?'

'I've no idea what you're talking about. But I have a question of my own.' Freya pointed towards the cow, as it came closer. 'Are those udders, or balls?'

'Balls!' Glenn yelled. 'Run!'

The beast bellowed, then, and gave chase, at horrendous speed. Freya tore off, the distance to the next stile closing rapidly, the fast pace no problem at all for her in her lightweight hillwalking shoes, even with the sodden ground. She glanced back at Glenn. He had fallen behind. While he kept his back straight and pistoned his arms, his gait was almost comically slow, as if he ran through treacle up to his waist.

The bull bellowed again. It was bearing down on him fast. There was a good couple of hundred yards' grace between them, but that was shortening, and fast.

Freya ran back. 'Give me the backpack.'

'No, carry on…'

'Give me the backpack, you berk!'

Glenn shook his head. 'Go on, get away. I'll be fine.'

'You'll be turned into a frigging shish kebab. I'm faster – give it to me. Life and death, here, mate. Don't argue. I'm fitter.' Without waiting for a reply, she snatched the rucksack off one shoulder. He sloped his shoulders to allow her to take the weight. Then they both took off. She still outpaced him until they reached the stile.

'No arguments – after you,' he said.

She didn't argue. She went up the stile, hurling the

backpack over onto the other side of the field. Only then she saw the bull, and it was too close, fifty feet, less, its eyes bloodshot and bulging. *I get it now, bullseye*, she thought, as she reached for Glenn, his face stricken, as he placed one foot on the bottom rung of the stile.

'You've got to jump!' she screamed. 'Jump!'

His hands locked with hers, the bull bellowed, a sound she felt in the core of her chest and down her spine, like a thunderclap, and Glenn leapt, his feet scrabbling, as the bull collided with the wall with a terrible crunch.

As they fell, the physics of it seemed all wrong, as if the rest of the planet had crashed into the bull instead of the other way around, but it had missed, and Freya's backward momentum and Glenn's forward motion combined, sending them both tumbling over the stile and into the boggy ground.

They both lay side by side for a few seconds, breathing hard. They listened to the bull's rage as it gored the wall, again and again.

'Still alive?' Freya said.

'Yep.'

'Nothing broken?'

'Not physically. Mentally, maybe.' Glenn sat up, and checked inside the rucksack. 'I'm going to clock that up as a close shave.'

'When this is over, I am going to get the biggest, bloodiest steak in history.' Freya got up and helped him to his feet. She was muddy, but unbloodied. So was he. He'd even managed to keep his glasses. 'I hope that we haven't missed another sign, saying, "The Field Of Many Bulls",' she said, scanning the horizon for more beasts.

'Me too,' he replied. 'I tell you what I've discovered today – I'm not the outdoor type.'

'Nah, me neither. I'll stick to cities, I think.'

Glenn shouldered the rucksack, holding the small of his back and wincing. 'At least we answered your question from earlier.'

'Which one?'

'The one about how fast I can get over the wall.'

'Shall we check out this scary tree now?'

'With luck.'

They turned towards the many-armed shadow on the horizon.

16

The oak was coming into bud, but nothing about that scene or that tree suggested springtime, or rebirth, or any of the benefits of the season. It was an ugly tree, spectacular enough to take a picture of, but old, stunted and bloated.

'No prizes for guessing why they call it the Hanging Oak,' Freya said.

'Think it was even more obvious about one hundred years ago. They cut off all the branches they used to dangle folk from.'

'This whole place is a bit *Wuthering Heights*.' Freya shivered, and gazed out across the bleak, uncultivated ground, bordered as far as the eye could see by a drystone wall up a slight incline. Thankfully, there were no animals, angry or otherwise, to be seen anywhere. They had just about recovered from their wildlife encounter – or at least, they had got their breath back.

Glenn dropped the rucksack, keeping it supported upright between his knees. When he unzipped the top, and began to withdraw a long, clean wooden handle, just for a second, Freya thought he was going to pull out an axe.

Instead, the head of a brand-new shovel appeared,

gleaming like a freshly minted silver coin. He tossed it on the ground, and began to withdraw something else, a long black plastic-coated stick.

Freya indicated the shovel. 'We going to dig this entire field?'

'I've got a horrible feeling we might have to. There's another one in here, hold on…' He pulled out a second, identical shovel. Then he began to fit the components of the other object. A large, flat disc at the bottom told Freya what it was.

'It's a pun,' she said. 'Test your mettle. He meant, test for metal. A metal detector.'

Glenn nodded, and a cheeky monkey grin spread across his face. 'Got to be honest – I've wanted an excuse to buy one of these for years.' The metal detector didn't look particularly high-tech, once it was assembled. The casing was beige, and apart from a digital control panel at the top, it might have been from the 1980s.

Freya watched as Glenn focused on the LCD display, a laser beam blue glow reflecting off the surface of his spectacles. 'Farmer going to be OK with this, yeah?'

'There's some dispute over who owns this field – nothing's been planted here, and animals aren't allowed in to graze, either. Stretches back to the days they put the tree back there to good use.'

'That probably makes it more likely someone will come over here and bust our chops for digging it up.'

Glenn shrugged. 'Probably.'

'And what's your plan for when that happens?'

'I'll say that you're an undercover cop.'

She laughed at that. 'When do I get a turn on the detector?'

'I guess we can swap over at half-time.'

'Just sweeping this whole field? Any ideas what we're looking for?'

'I should think that's obvious.'

It wasn't totally obvious to Freya, so she remained silent. 'Anything I can do to help, then?'

'Take some pictures of me in action. Left hand side's my best. I'll do a pout for you.' He walked over to the furthest corner of the field, the detector over his shoulder. She did take a picture of this, on her camera. On a whim, she took another in black and white, taking care to get the tree in. Black and white suited the tree a lot better; in silhouette its bulges and blemishes lost their texture, became less threatening.

'I thought they hanged people at crossroads?' Freya said.

Glenn's reply was distant. 'This used to be a crossroads, years ago. The road's been swallowed up, but you can just about make out the impression of where it was. It's like having an old railway – you can still see where the embankments are. Same with the road. There used to be a town, round about here. All gone now. Just the odd bit of wreckage poking out of the ground. Rubble. Farmer bought it all over.'

'Right. Whereabouts is the road, exactly?'

Glenn signed, and shouldered the metal detector. 'The tree's at the crossroads, as you say. It's in the middle. The road splits three ways.'

Freya walked over to a crease in the ground. It was only noticeable from a certain angle, but there was a definite scar in the earth. 'I think I can make it out... Looks like three roads, criss-crossing round about the tree.'

'Yes,' Glenn said, impatiently.

'So, three forks, then. Or tines, if we're being picky. And you usually are.'

He stopped.

'Our mystery man said, "the Middle Fork",' Freya continued. 'That refers to what this place is called. I get that. But maybe he was trying to make things easy for us. He wants us to find something. I don't think he'd want us to take all day about it.'

Glenn stopped what he was doing, and came over to join her. 'Fair comment. Let's see what we find. There's always the chance that it's a hoax. Someone who knows you and read the paper… It's a possibility. Part of me hopes that's all it is, and this is a wild goose chase. If it isn't, a multiple murderer on the loose knows where you live.' At Freya's stricken face, he raised a hand. 'Sorry.'

'I've had it in my mind all along. Don't apologise. I just don't know what I'm going to do about it.'

'Let's see what turns up.' He actually patted her, once, on the shoulder. Quickly, he said: 'Right. I deduce that we should be following the middle fork of the three, as it approaches the tree. We should probably start where this quote unquote, middle fork, reaches the tree, then travel along the road. That would be the simplest place to start looking. Was that what you meant?'

'You read my mind.'

They did so. Up close, the tree was even uglier. There was a bole fashioned in the middle, a deep, dark portal about seven feet above ground.

'Reckon he meant that hole?' Freya said.

'Best to check.' A sweep of the bole revealed nothing.

Freya pondered a moment. 'Maybe he left a clue in there? Seems an obvious place, if he's being obvious.'

Glenn swivelled his head towards her. 'I'm not putting my hand in that hole for a million pounds. But you be my guest.'

The detector beeped a couple of times, and they had to get to work with the shovels. Freya's back ached, along with the soles of her feet as she kicked the blade into the earth. All they dislodged were worms, lots of them, and bottle tops.

'This may yet take a while,' Glenn said, gulping down water. 'Maybe he's not making it that easy for us.'

'You have to ask... whenever we find what we're looking for, assuming we haven't done this for no good reason... what does he want?'

'I have wondered what his game is. Assuming he's the Woodcutter. Assuming he's a real person.'

Freya rested her elbow on the handle of the shovel. 'What's that supposed to mean?'

'I'm just being honest with you. Just speculating. You've come to me with an actual cloak-and-dagger story. If it turned out to be bollocks, many people would not find this surprising. I don't know exactly what happened. I'm just going by what you said. For all I know, you just want to get me out here on my own.'

Freya straightened up. 'And, for all I know, you might know more about this than you're letting on.'

'Excuse me?' He looked genuinely nettled, which was pleasing to her.

'I mean, how did you get home the other night? At the pub?'

He shrugged. 'Taxi.'

'Or maybe you followed me. For all I know, it was you.'

'Realms of fantasy.' He looked pained, though.

'Just being honest with you.'

'Well, let's see what turns up. As you say, it's just an idea. We could have put two and two together, and got…'

The metal detector shrieked. They both flinched. He had been passing it over the path, absent-mindedly. It emitted a low hum, except for when it had picked up the bottle tops. But those had been mild pings; this was a full-on alarm.

Glenn fixed the position, checking the readings. 'Something substantial down there, for sure.'

'This is very symmetrical. Look at the field, the wall, the tree. I've got a feeling we're on the right lines.'

They began to dig. The grassy clumps and the weeds came up, as did the stony ground. Bizarrely, the soil reminded Freya of cake mix, not entirely unappealing, if you discounted the beetles and worms who twisted away from the shovel blades' crude intrusions. Something in Freya wanted to delve her hands into it.

They soon found what they were looking for.

'What's that?' Freya said, indicating something solid.

'Wood,' Glenn said, simply.

'Surely it would have rotted down there?'

'It's been treated. Looks like some kind of lacquer. Watertight, anyway.' He ticked a fingernail against it.

They began to uncover it.

'This is it, isn't it?' Freya said, quietly. Almost a statement, not a question.

Glenn said nothing, but his face betrayed some excitement,

his eyes quick. He took several photographs of each stage. Freya felt only a sense of dread.

The end of the handle had been angled downwards, as if piled into the earth some time ago and left there. It was a long, strong shaft, as long as the handles on the shovels they used to turn the earth. The going got easier the further down they went, although it was more moist, messier. Their shoes and trousers became mired with rank soil, and the smell of it turned Freya's stomach.

'This is it,' Glenn whispered, at length.

The blade still looked new. It was thick, red-stained; the colour was like a lightning bolt in that drab surrounding, vivid as blood.

'Jesus H Christ and his holy chariot,' Freya said.

'Don't touch it,' Glenn said. 'Not with your fingers.' He put on some clear plastic gloves. Then he began to dig around it, carefully.

It was an axe, of course. Not new; and it had been there for quite some time. It stayed at an angle of about forty-five degrees to the line of the horizon.

'It's stuck in something,' Glenn said. 'Wait a second…'

He reached into the earth, and began to lift out some of the muck with his hands. One great, fat earthworm squirmed clear of his fingers. He cried out in disgust, and Freya was about to make a remark about being spooked about a simple worm. Then she saw what he had cleared away.

The blade of the axe was stuck fast in something brown and off-yellow, something that glared at both of them with caked eye-sockets. It was split cleanly down the middle, and thankfully they were spared the sight of its eternal grin. But there could be no doubt that they were looking at a skull.

17

In the shower a few days later, Freya noticed that some dirt still clung to some parts of her hands. It had wanted to cling to her, to burrow in deep in the grooves and loops. She had craved her bed when she got home, but now the shadows were alive, and every silence felt like a killer in every nook of the flat, holding his breath.

The video app call startled her, and she was stunned to see that her hand was properly shaking. She had to tense her forearm to the point of pain to calm down the tremor.

Glenn's face appeared as an abstract series of blocks, pink and brown and blond. This building block effect merged quite beautifully with his glasses, before settling into a clear, if not sharp image on Freya's tablet screen. He was wearing a collar and tie – stark white slit with red – but seemed to be in his front room. A table lamp provided some pleasant ambient light over one shoulder.

'How'd it go, then?' she asked.

'Short answer: they know I'm a liar. It's not the first time I've been interviewed by the cops, but this is the first time they think I did something *wrong*.'

Freya frowned. 'Have you done something wrong? I thought you'd done them a really, really big favour.'

'I'm not telling them the whole truth. And I'm doing this for you. They're suspicious about how I came by the information.'

'Think about it. If you were to say that the daughter of the man who they put in jail for being the Woodcutter had contacted you, and just after that, someone left her a note, telling her where to find one of the bodies… It wouldn't seem like the truth. Would it?'

'It is the truth, though. And it was a mistake not to tell them. I shouldn't have let you talk me into it.'

'They would draw a line between me contacting my dad, and this information. It would keep him in jail. I don't think the tip came from him, or one of his pen pals. It's the real killer – someone who wants my dad kept in jail. That's the clincher, for me. I think it's the real killer. I know we're withholding something from them. But I'm not revealing that just yet.'

'He might have left some traces… witnesses, CCTV… something, surely.'

'I went back to the forest… the arrows are gone. Totally cut out. The bark is shredded – so it's a fresh wound, but it doesn't look regular, as if some letters had been carved. You wouldn't know it was there. Must have gone round with vinegar or sugar soap. Sneaky bastard. For all I know, he did it minutes after I saw it. Wouldn't surprise me.'

'There's the other problem. You.'

'What do you mean?'

'Security.'

'Let me worry about that. Anyway… I would've thought you would be happy. You got your scoop. Was the picture of the skull really necessary on your site?'

'Veritas. It was as it was. The papers paid a fortune for the pictures.'

'Good for you,' Freya said, curtly.

'Hey, I'm in business like anyone else.'

Freya resisted the temptation to hit the off switch. 'Not sure I like that attitude.'

'You seemed to like it just fine when you wrote an article for the *Salvo*.'

'That was different.'

'Not really. Anyway, we can go fifty-fifty if you like, on the profits. So long as you take fifty-fifty on the heat.'

'The heat?' she snorted. 'Unless you put that skeleton there, there's no heat. You've watched too many movies. You found a body. You told them about it. They've got something to work on.'

'You weren't there, in the interview room. The SIO's name was Connor Tamm – same guy who tailed you on the farm track. Detective Inspector Tamm. Wavy hair. Streaks of white in it, like a superhero in a comic. Still looked far too young to be in the police. He was smart, though. No underestimating him. I had to rehearse what I was going to say a dozen times. He took me back and forth. I was throwing tells and tics all over the place. I couldn't stop it. He got shouty at one point, him and the other officer.'

'Do you think they believed you?'

'As I said – no chance. I guess they spot liars a mile away.'

'God. I'd hate that. Thank you.' Freya had not wanted to be involved with the police – had been adamant that she wanted no part of the conversation, after Glenn had decided to tell them about the body. She knew it was a risk to her father – she saw the way it was being gamed out. How she was being played, in order to keep Gareth Solomon in prison, even to allow for a fresh investigation. They didn't have much time to get their stories straight. They admitted, however, that they had separately pre-figured something out just in the off chance they were going to find something significant, and the resultant pooling of information went like this:

Glenn had long wanted to explore the field near the Hanging Oak, as he was an enthusiast about all things horrible and murderous. This had the feeling of the Lord's honest truth, as Glenn noted. All manner of things were reputedly buried there from the days when people would gather to watch someone have their neck stretched – coins, buckles, things that the plough would ordinarily have turned up, except the land was in dispute and uncultivated for more than a hundred years.

The part which no one believed, and neither Glenn nor Freya expected them to believe, was that, a matter of days after the Woodcutter had appeared in the papers, while the man convicted of being said killer was appealing against his conviction, one of his missing victims' bodies should show up. And not only that, but it would be uncovered by a blogger who they regarded as an irritant and sensationalist at best.

'Any thoughts over who the body belonged to?'

'I couldn't say whether the skull was male or female. I don't have the forensic skills to differentiate between the two on sight, though I do know one or two people who could help. But it wasn't really the skull that got my interest. It was the axe.'

'That's for sure. The way you behaved, it's as if you'd

found the bloody Lost Ark. The spear of destiny, or something.'

'The spear of Longinus, you may be referring to. The one that supposedly pierced Christ's side.'

'Whatever, Glenn.' She prepared to bite deep into a slice of toast; then thought better of it. In truth, she had been off her food. During a stint working in a care home, she had known death; had seen it close up, so many times that it became less scary. But the skull in the earth was something else, something darker. She'd slept with the lights on since that day.

'I had to tell them that I touched the handle,' Glenn said. 'The minute you touch it, you could invalidate evidence.'

'Or make you a suspect.'

'Good work killing someone before I was born, you have to say.'

'You were saying? About the victim?'

'I think it was Max Dilworth. The ex-special forces guy.'

'Special forces?' Freya said. 'I thought he was in the Royal Artillery.'

'That's what everyone wants you to think. He passed selection. They don't advertise it.' 'How did you know… wait. Sources.'

He tapped his forehead. 'Exactly right.'

They hadn't seen any clothes that might indicate who the person in the field was; they weren't even sure if there were any other body parts down there. All they had was those two mud-encrusted eyes, gazing up at them. In the five known Woodcutter cases, Max Dilworth had been the anomaly. He was the outlier, the only male victim of the five. There was still some doubt over how he had disappeared, with many believing that he had been kidnapped by the IRA, still very much in operation at the time, although this had been strenuously denied by the Republicans. Every other aspect of Max Dilworth's disappearance tied in with the Woodcutter's work, though. A man out on a run, on a lonely road (this time a canal bank), vanished without trace, with some people reporting a black transit van in the area.

'What's your reasoning?'

'The dates and locations tie up – he was my main candidate. Remember, when we looked at the locations? The Hanging Oak is the closest point to where Dilworth was abducted. There's something weird about the fact the axe was left there, though. It's a message, almost. Or a taunt. The police were meant to find that, I think. Over time.'

'Not sure that makes sense. June Caton-Bell was the last victim – that's what led them to arrest my dad. Why would he leave the axe somewhere, and then kill someone else?'

'I have to admit, that's puzzled me. But there it is. The Woodcutter was a secretive killer – that's why we only ever found one body. Maybe he was getting bolder, the more victims he had. A natural escalation. You see it in other killers. Maybe he was getting off on the attention from the press, once they got wind of what he was up to. Max Dilworth has always been the odd one out, though. The theory I buy into is that he set himself a challenge – he enjoyed the chase, and the thrill of catching them. An ex-forces guy would have been a scalp to take. Then once he catches up with them, there's the frenzy, the overkill. It's odd that there's not much of a sexual element, or doesn't appear to be. This is a different kind of sadism. It's weird.'

'He got off on the kill, though. And the fear.'

Glenn was pensive for a moment. Then he smiled. 'You've got me doing it, now.'

'Doing what?'

'Talking about the Woodcutter in the abstract. As if he's not your dad.'

'You said it yourself,' she said, a trifle defensively. 'Be open and rational. Admit to every possibility. One of these is that my dad was telling the truth. That he is in jail for something he didn't do. That the Woodcutter is still out there, and he's getting in touch with me. After I got in touch with my dad. Maybe it's just self-preservation. Maybe it's something personal. Whoever it was, wanted me to get in touch with the police, that's clear. But there's something missing. Some connection.'

'I know.' Glenn scratched the back of his neck. 'There are so many rogue elements, here. Something missing in every theory. Something that casts doubt on what we think we know. A few things have to happen now. First, we've got to find Carol Ramirez. She's been difficult to trace. Changed her name, I think. I've exhausted my sources. Second, we need to speak to Bernard Galvin. Now he's easy to find. But not to speak to.'

'This "we" you speak of… We definitely partners, yes?'

'If you like.'

'So that means, we share our leads.'

'If you like. It also means that you tell me whatever you're planning to do with the papers.'

'That's different. That stuff's personal – we didn't investigate that.'

'So far as I'm aware you didn't do any research on the Hanging Oak, anything like that…'

'Bugger off! I gave you the tip. I had the contact. You did nothing. A bloody internet search! Took you all of two minutes, if that.'

'Fifty-fifty, then. That's the way it has to be.'

She nodded, reluctantly. 'All right. Maybe we could write a book.'

'I was thinking that. But there's one other thing we need to do: make sure you're safe.'

'You don't have to worry about me.'

'I would stay somewhere else, if you can. Short-term. If you were in contact with the Woodcutter, he knows who you are, thanks to the newspaper article. That means he knows where you live.'

'Think about it, Glenn. If he'd meant to do me some harm, he would have done it already. He wouldn't have been dropping me cryptic clues.'

'I still think you should tell the police about that.'

'I'm not approaching the police with this, now. They've got what they need – something they've been looking for, for years. Whoever was down there, their poor family will get to have a decent burial.'

'We're talking about a psychopathic killer. Stay safe. Please.'

'You don't have to worry about me. I can take care of myself.' She didn't sound too sure of herself; the old diffidence had crept in. 'Anyway. I've got things to think about. And I also have someone to speak to, today.'

'Who?'

'My dad. Speak next time.' Freya cut the connection, sat back in her seat, and yawned. Best get to work.

Then she heard… not quite a creak. More of a shift; a someone light on their feet, disturbing rough carpeting, say.

Rough carpeting, like the oatmeal stuff tacked to the hallway outside.

The hair at the back of her neck roiled. She stood up from the seat, rigid. She held her breath and listened.

Nothing. She waited, ten seconds, thirty, a minute, perhaps more. Then nothing.

She took a step or two towards the door. Then she heard it again. A shift. Not someone upstairs. Not mice, not the neighbours through the walls. *Someone padding around, outside the front door*.

But it was too subtle a sound to be absolutely sure. Freya had her finger on the "emergency call" button; then told herself off. *Imagining things. Too much going on at the moment. Dead bodies and God knows what else. Plus my dad's in jail for murder – fancy that.*

Nonetheless she crept through the hallway towards the door, and slid back the cover on the fish-eye lens.

Now if a face had loomed into view at that particular moment, Freya would have screamed her head off. She might have left her skin, her body behind, and soared free. But no horror movie face appeared, and better yet, the weird bubble of peripheral vision showed there was no one at either side of the corridor, either. In order for someone to be hiding outside her front door, they'd have to be hiding behind the door at the end of the corridor. And that was too far for them to run, before Freya could get back into her front door.

Freya crossed over to the coat rack, pausing for a moment on sight of the old jackets lined up there, which she hadn't had the chance to get rid of, yet. Then she put on her own jacket, checked the security lens again, then unlocked the door.

The instant she did so, the security door to the left burst open and a spindly man sprinted down the hall, too fast to focus on, like a spider suddenly breaking cover from beneath a couch.

A man. Here, now, my flat.

Him!

She screamed, her hand scrambling on the door handle. She got it open and ran back in; but before she could slam the door shut, a foot blocked it over her threshold.

Mick Harvie was right in her face, on the doorstop, his face set in a snarl, and close enough to feel his warm breath and spit on her cheeks.

'Well, there she is,' he growled. 'There she is.'

18

Harvie's snarl faded a little. His eyes darted, taking in Freya's hair, her make-up.

'Hey – Jesus. What have you done to your hair?'

Freya leaned back, taking her weight on her standing leg, and then stabbed a vicious kick at Harvie's mid-section.

The effect was extraordinary – he barked out a cry of pain that echoed down the communal stairwell, buckled in the middle and slammed backwards into the whitewashed wall at his back.

He had to steady himself against the wall to stop himself pitching forward onto the floor, knees sagging. He clutched his hip where she'd hit him, his mossy chin agape. 'What the fuck?'

Freya was back in her flat, her reflexes utterly in control. She had turned the key and thrown the chain over the door without consciously processing that she had actually done it, then placed her eye against the fish-eye spyhole. A distorted Mick Harvie lurched forward, a caricature of his own bearded face, stretched out across her entire visual field.

'What are you playing at? I came to talk!'

'You could have phoned me. How did you get into this building?'

Harvie fought for breath; the blood had drained from his face; he spat on the floor. She rather hoped he was sick, notwithstanding the inconvenience of cleaning up after him. 'I followed the postie in. I had to make sure you wouldn't hang up on me. Or slam the door in my face. Or try to kick me in the balls!'

Freya heard the door across the way opening up, and the elderly woman who lived there said, querulously: 'What's going on out there? Do you need to leave a parcel?'

Freya unlocked the door. 'Get back,' she said to Harvie, quietly. When he did so, Freya emerged from the doorway and lifted a hand to the frightened little face that appeared across the way. 'It's OK, Mrs Townsend. This is a friend of my mum's. Sorry to disturb you.'

'You never used to be this noisy!'

'I'm awfully sorry. We were just heading out.' She closed and locked the door behind her. 'You going to be OK there, Uncle Mick?'

He straightened back up, but it was clearly an effort. 'Fine,' he said, though not too convincingly.

'Take care, Mrs Townsend,' Freya said, waving. She stepped past Mick Harvie and opened the fire door, not waiting to see whether he followed, or whether Mrs Townsend had closed her door.

'Never do that to me again,' he growled in her ear. 'Understand? Never.'

She smiled over her shoulder. 'Never spring out on me again – or you'll get it worse. Got it, Uncle Mick?'

'Where we going?'

'A very safe, very public place.'

The playpark across the road was populated by a twitchy flock of mothers and fathers taking their pre-schoolers out for some precarious activities on top of see-saws, roundabouts and safety swings. It also had two park benches, side by side. Freya had been quite clear that Mick Harvie should sit on one, while she should sit on the other, although she began to pace the moment he sat down.

His cheeks pinched tight in discomfort as he did so. 'Where did you learn the fancy skills? You into martial arts?'

'No. I went to aikido when I was nine for a few weeks. I thought it was too rough, would you believe. Lot of nasty boys there, who didn't like me. But my mum told me it was a good idea to learn one move really well. She was right. It's like mastering a card trick. Some guy tried to break into the pub, one night. I got him as he was climbing through the broken window. He got off his mark, quick enough.'

'I believe it.'

'Don't be keeping me in suspense, Mick. What do you want?'

'First of all – I take it you've heard about the body they found the other day?'

'Yeah. Couldn't miss it, could I? They had an expert on to talk about it on the news. Said there's every chance it's one of the missing bodies in the Woodcutter case.'

He nodded. 'Yeah. That little twerp on the website found it, somehow. The guy who does the podcasts. Red Ink? Something like that?'

'Yeah. An amateur, or something.'

'Seems a bit of a coincidence, doesn't it?' He squinted at her through the late morning sunlight. 'He happened to be looking for buried treasure, and he finds something connected to the Woodcutter. A few days after the Woodcutter appears in the press, again.'

Freya shrugged. 'I can't control events.'

'Maybe you can't, but someone can. Have you spoken to Glenn Allander in the past few weeks?'

'None of your business, Mick. I thought you wanted to talk about something? I know they've found a body. I know it might be Max Dilworth.'

'It is Max Dilworth.' He regarded her evenly. 'And I'm pretty sure you've spoken to Glenn Allander.'

'Big deal. You my dad or something?'

'Nope. I know who your dad is. And so does everybody else. Make no mistake about it.' His smile faded. 'You've changed the hair – probably a good move, given the hassle you might be about to have. As close to a disguise as you can get. Not one hundred per cent sure blonde suits you, but that's just my opinion. But without that eye make-up, you look so much like him it's *freaky*.'

'Sorry for existing. You got any more tabloid advice for me? Any makeover tips? Shall I wear a nice short skirt? Unbutton my top, maybe?' She gestured towards some bushes, visible through the waist-high fencing about one hundred yards away. 'Got someone stationed in there? Candid shots? Should I wear a *very* revealing outfit? Don't waste my time. Get to the point, Mick.'

'The reason I came to see you was to warn you that I've heard some rumblings from my sources at the police.'

'Rumblings? Was it happy hour at the doughnut shop?'

'There's something about to break in the Woodcutter case. Cold case review team have been going nuts. It was worth passing on, I think.'

'And what do you want in return for that?'

'I've come to make you an offer. Another feature – guaranteed two-page spread at one of the nationals.'

She sighed. 'I'm not doing this for big offers, Mick. I'm doing this because my dad's my last living relative, and I think the courts, the police, and the press let him down. I wish you'd understand that.'

'The nationals have been in contact, though. I know that.' He grinned.

'You don't know everything. When I mentioned you to the guy at the *Sentinel*, he burst out laughing. Said he thought you were in the retirement home for embittered hacks. What can he mean?'

'Wowzers!' He cackled. 'With a bit of that chutzpah, you could be a star on the nationals!'

Freya stared at her feet, feeling colour rise to her cheeks. 'I'm sorry. That was totally uncalled for. He didn't say that. I didn't mean to be so nasty.'

He dismissed her apology with an impatient wave of the hand. 'The *Sentinel*, you say? Half those clowns don't know they're born. They're hardly out of school. Bit like yourself.' He could not stop a sneer breaking free of his beard. 'Think they can control the world through a computer terminal. Get their stories that way, too. Start to see life through pixels, not flesh and blood. But life isn't quite automated yet. It isn't all emails and social media. Most of that's a lie – or a misunderstanding, at best. To get to the truth, you have to speak to people. Get their confidence. That means getting off your arse and talking to them. Face-to-face. Not on a screen.'

'So, when you stalked me and waited outside my front door this morning... what was that, Mick? A charm offensive?'

'I've told you my reasoning. You might have ignored me. And at the end of the day – you're very interesting. But you're not the story. The Woodcutter is the story. He's the be-all and end-all. Whoever he might be.'

'You seemed pretty sure the Woodcutter was my dad, the last time we met. Now you're being vague. Something changed your mind?'

Harvie took a flask of water from his jacket pocket, unscrewed the cap and took a sip. Somewhat bizarrely, he offered it to her; she shook her head.

'Too early for me, Mick. Not opening time yet.'

'It's water,' he said, without a trace of humour. He screwed the cap back on. 'I'll say it again. Your dad's a son of a bitch. He's not right. And he chopped up June Caton-Bell, and the rest of them. I know it. But he's got wriggle room, legally. And his appeal has got the cops spooked. That was before the axe and the skeleton turned up in the field.'

'Nobody mentioned an axe,' Freya said. 'Just remains. They held that back.'

'I mentioned an axe. I've got sources, remember? They found an axe. Added to the appeal, something's bothering them. Particularly Bernard Galvin.'

'The copper who put my dad away, you mean?'

'One of many. But yeah, him in particular. He took the press conferences. He got his big ball face in the cameras outside court. A good copper, as I say. Not someone you want to cross. But fair. And he got his man, no doubt about that.'

'So, what's spooked him? What do you know?'

'You up for doing another feature?'

'Maybe. But that means you tell me everything you know.'

His mock-innocent face was one of the most slappable Freya had ever seen in real life. 'Me?'

'Yes, you. You held things back from me, then sold them on the back of my article. I don't care about the money. But you ripped me off last time. Spare me the patter.'

'You agreed to the piece in the *Salvo*. I didn't mention any other paper. Or what I knew.'

'Your word for the day is "disingenuous", Mick.'

'And yours is "experience". You've learned something. So – I promise to share the goods, and you give me some words. Deal?'

'Deal.' They shook on it. 'Now – what have you got to tell me?'

'Something of interest. Something you might know. And something Glenn Allander doesn't know. If he did, he'd have splattered it all over that miserable website of his, the way he does with everything else. See, this is the thing with the geeks – they don't know what to put out there, and what to hold back. They just spew everything out. There's no nuance. No control. Everything's for show and effect. But there's restraint in the press. You might not think it, but there is. We have a duty of care. Normally when I say that, people burst out laughing, and point to cases where...'

'What's the new stuff you've got for me, Mick? Be quick. I have things to do today.'

'There's a site of interest to the cops. It's not new; from way back. I never knew why. But Bernard Galvin wants it opened up again. Wants the cold case team to look at it. Somewhere he was interested in when one of the other victims vanished. Somewhere a black van had been seen. Near an abandoned quarry. Nothing was found, but he wants it opened up. He still thinks one of the missing bodies is there. Given the timeline, it's probably Anne-Marie Kittrick.'

Freya contained her impatience, but only just. 'Whereabouts?'

'You'll like this.' He smiled. 'It's a ghost town. I'll send you the location. You can check it out, if you like.'

'You coming with us?'

'Not this time. I've got one or two tips of my own I want to follow up. Could be a dead end. Might not be a dead end. Anyway. Stay tuned, Freya.'

He made his way off – limping slightly. Mixed feelings, Freya thought. There's a man who deserves a kick in the balls, all right. Then she remembered lashing out. She remembered his face contorting in surprise and pain. That wasn't her. Martial arts or no martial arts. She covered her face and sighed.

She would have to ask her dad more about him.

19

Gareth Solomon seemed so jocular that Freya would have sworn he was on something. Rather than a bullet-headed wrestler gone to seed, he now more closely resembled the jolly older male relative at a family barbecue he would have been in an alternate reality.

One-way banter filtered through the air as he was buzzed through the security door; it wasn't clear if the guard accompanying him gave any reply. Solomon's eyes were compressed into tight-packed lines of mirth. That was, until he saw her.

'Whoa. What have you done to your hair?'

'I had to make a change or two. The press. Nosy people in general. You know how it is.'

'God, that's some difference. I mean the mascara and the whole Morticia Addams thing, it was a good look… All said and done, I prefer a blonde, that's true.'

'Thanks…' She took a deep breath. Her mouth didn't want to form the word. She felt herself blushing. This was a risk… And yet, it felt like the right thing to say, so she said: '…Dad.'

He grinned. 'It'll take a bit of getting used to, this.'

'Being a human?'

'Well put! Being a father's close enough, I guess. I didn't have the best role models in that regard, as I already told you.'

'You heard he died?'

'So they told me. Second or third-hand. I heard he died while I was inside. Someone passed me a death notice clipped out the local paper. "After a long illness," it said. Cancer, I hope. He never saw the inside of a prison for what he did. No idea what happened to the brothers and sisters, to this day – after I ended up in care. Never bothered to keep in touch, and they certainly didn't want to keep in touch with me. Especially since I ended up in here. The papers said I had the classic journey – from the firm hand of daddy to minor crime, then bigger crimes, and finally – a great big one. Allegedly.'

After a pause, Freya said: 'I'm sorry that happened to you.'

Solomon shrugged, then said in a startlingly camp voice: 'Over it, girlfriend.' He paused for a response. When it didn't arrive, he said: 'Is that still something people say on the outside?'

'It's not quite the same language, but I can work out what it means through the context.'

'That patter's twenty-five years old, I guess. As old as you are.' He cocked his head at her, and narrowed his eyes. 'There's something you want to ask me. Spill it. Go.'

'I want to follow up on what I mentioned last time. I want to talk a little bit about some of the victims.'

'Victims.' He nodded intently, and faded out for a second or two. 'OK. Victims. Whose victims, exactly?'

'The Woodcutter's.'

He leaned back in his chair and pinched his nose. The silence that followed seemed to portend a detonation of sorts, and she steeled herself for it – as did the guard over his shoulder, who braced himself for an outburst, or worse. But instead, Solomon almost whispered: 'And why would I want to talk about someone else's victims?'

'Because you were linked to each abduction. I want to hear you talk about why it wasn't you.'

'Retrace my steps? OK. I can do that. I know it off the top of my head by now. Could sit an exam. Hit me – who was first? Anne-Marie Kittrick? Underpass girl?'

'That's right.'

'I drove over that underpass four times, two days before she vanished. Apparently on the first day, she was on a training run. But the time of the training run doesn't quite match the time I drove past. On the second time, she wasn't there. The reason I drove over that underpass was because I was ferrying car parts from a garage to a go-karting racetrack, would you believe, fourteen miles down the bendy little A-road that fed into the main road. I never clapped eyes on her.'

'What about the day she vanished?'

'Nowhere near the place... in fact, I might have been going to see your mum. That would be about right.'

'No record of you anywhere, though.'

'There is, though. I had to take some repaired computer equipment all the way down the south coast, starting the morning after she was killed. Bit of a stretch that I did it, made a pick-up then drove all the way down, isn't it?'

'But you were placed close to her. You could have spotted her and stalked her, couldn't you?'

'I didn't.' He stared into her eyes. 'It's trumped up. It wasn't me.'

'Now… Coleen Arden.'

'Oh yeah. Good-looking girl. I saw enough photos of her. In the papers, you know. Looked like someone on *Coronation Street* or *EastEnders*. Wasn't me, before you ask.'

'You had checked into a hotel close to the train station, which was the last place she was seen before she vanished on the Downs.'

'And I had checked in with a woman. Police know who she was, and spoke to her.'

'She said she was blind drunk the night it happened and can't swear if you were there or not. No CCTV cameras showing you going in or out, back then. You parked on the street.'

'But I was there, and I woke up next to her the next morning. It's true she was drunk. She was like that. Next.'

'Max Dilworth. Tyre tracks, near the canal track. Van found burnt out – similar to the one you drove. You didn't have any work that week.'

'But not the one I drove. I didn't own any other transit vans. I reckon that boy was killed by the IRA – nothing to do with the Woodcutter. I think the Woodcutter was into girls. If the police have got anything linking Max Dilworth to the Woodcutter cases, they haven't made it clear to me or anyone connected to my case. Fishing trip, that one. You want my opinion, the security services are embarrassed about it. Pin the tail on the serial killer.'

'Danielle Pearson. The wheatfield. Dog walker. You were helping drive tractors on a farm.'

'A farm... fifty miles away. And it was hard work on those farms, let me tell you. Some rough boys work there. I didn't go back there. I lasted a couple of weeks then moved on.'

'Yes... They couldn't trace the men you worked with, on the evening she vanished.'

'They were casual workers, backpackers, seasonal bods... drifters. I couldn't tell you their names, confidently. One of them might have been from Lithuania. I had nothing to do with it.'

'And June Caton-Bell.' Freya folded her arms. 'The night you were with Carol Ramirez.'

He shrugged. 'I don't have anything to say about that. It wasn't me – that much I can tell you. I can't say anything more. I can't say anything about Carol, either. So don't ask.'

'It's the one they got you for.'

'I didn't do it. That's all I'll say.' He smiled.

'You seem in a good mood, talking about dead girls, I have to say.'

Solomon leaned forward, bracing his elbows on the table. He thrust his chin downwards, and cast his eyes upwards. 'Aren't I just? I'm bouncing up and down about the stuff I read in the papers. So, why don't you fill me in – you might know more than me. Skulls and axes in a field, would you believe it? The cat is among the pigeons. How'd you find out about that?'

'Someone tipped me off.'

'How? If you don't mind my asking.'

Freya smiled, but his unblinking stare caused the hairs to stand up on her arms and the back of her neck. *If I'm wrong... This might have been the last thing some of them saw. Maybe it's what his expression was, right before he snatched them. Before he started snarling.* 'Anonymous tip-off. You didn't have anything to do with it, did you?'

'Much as I would love to pretend to be an evil puppet master pulling the strings from in here... Nope. Not me. It was the real Woodcutter. You must suspect that.'

'I'm keeping an open mind.'

'It's him, don't doubt it. Now... What does he want with you, daughter of mine?'

'You want my opinion... He's seen you in the papers. He wants to draw attention back to himself. Maybe he wants to come out of retirement. I'm not sure. It draws the scent away from you, though. Helps your case.'

'Maybe.' He drummed his fingers on the table. 'Anyway. Plod looking after you?'

'I guess.'

'You're in danger.'

'I know I'm in danger!' she blurted out. 'Sometimes I can't think about anything else! I've got a panic alarm set up in the house, since the bones were found in the field. The police say they've been patrolling, but... I can't be sure. They've been saying elsewhere the police haven't got money. They aren't investigating crimes. They can't post sentries at my door, exactly. Sorry.' She brushed a tear from the corner of her eye. 'It's been weird. It's been stressful. I know, it's been my fault... For getting involved. Sticking my nose in. I could have let it go, just kept it a secret. But it didn't feel like the right thing to do. It's not me as a person.'

He raised his hand. 'I'm sorry. Please stay safe – whoever it is out there, they might mean you harm, if what you say is right. Don't take chances. Maybe you shouldn't come here again.'

She shook her head. 'No. I've come too far for that.'

'They assigned a detective to you?'

'One has been in contact.'

'God help you if it's Bernie Galvin.' Solomon twitched, alarmingly. 'Seriously, try not to spend a lot of time alone. I don't want to find out I have a daughter, then find out I... don't.' He blinked, suddenly, then looked away. Solomon didn't look as if he was upset, exactly, just deeply uncomfortable. How does a psychopath process emotion? Can they process emotion? 'Anyway. Let's not lower the tone,' he continued. 'It's been a trail of good news this week. Sweet little crumbs.'

'You had some more good news?'

'Oh, you betcha. Glad tidings tickle my ears. We're in court soon. And I'm very, very confident I'll get a result. Could be that the next time we have a chinwag, I'll be a free man.' He paused. 'I mean, isn't that exciting? We could have a proper father-daughter relationship. Whatever that is.'

She felt an absurd feeling of warmth and contentment at these words – she struggled to keep it from her face. 'If you're cleared, then yes. We can have that. I'll do that for you. What're your glad tidings, then?'

'Well, ordinarily I'd be wary of opening my gob about anything in here, but... You promise not to tell?'

'Cross my heart. Hope to die.'

'It seems old Bernie Galvin's getting a bit worked up. Something's turned up. Well, apart from that dead guy with the axe in his skull. It seems that there's something they found in the grave alongside that jigsaw puzzle they found in the farmer's field. Something that led them to the old quarry. A place of interest, they call it. It seems that they might have found an old black van in there. One that might have been used in the Woodcutter cases. Yes. Must have been there a good while. Out in all the old caves and what have you. Surprised it hasn't rusted away to a shell. And you know the really strange thing about the black van they may or may not have found in the caves? It's got absolutely nothing to do with me.'

'You scrapped your black van. Not long before you were arrested.'

'That's right. See, I'm not a Mensa kid. I won't lie to you – I was very stupid, and also a bit panicky and desperate, when it turned out a witness had seen me creeping out of Carol Ramirez's house. And describing a black van. And June Caton-Bell turning up in those woods. So I took what I thought was a logical step. I had my black van scrapped. Got a mate of mine to do it. Pledged to put it in the crusher. Twenty quid, cash in hand. Owed me a favour. Except he wasn't that much of a mate, as he sang like a bird to the coppers right after it. Where things get really juicy is that Bernie Galvin claimed he turned up some evidence. Hair strands, he said, from June Caton-Bell. Only, June Caton-Bell wasn't anywhere near my old van in her life. Now, if the real black van should turn up in an old quarry, down the bottom of a shaft somewhere, and if there should be genuine evidence in there… Things might get a bit awkward for Bernie Galvin. Wouldn't you say?'

Freya remembered to breathe properly. She kept a smile fixed on her face. And she recalled Mick Harvie's warning:

'Your father's a liar. Remember that. Don't believe anything he says.'

'Carol Ramirez is an interesting character,' she said.

'Isn't she just? I thought so. You know, there was a time, I thought we might be soul mates. I hesitate to say that. No disrespect to your mother. I mean, I had a real connection with her, too, no denying that.'

'One that you broke immediately, once you got her pregnant.'

'Now, that hurts my feelings.' It didn't appear to have done this at all. He sighed, and folded his arms. 'Actually, yeah, you're right. Adult relationships – sometimes they're complicated. And sometimes, they're not.'

'So, you were with Carol Ramirez. You admit that. Strange that it was never mentioned during your trial.'

Solomon clucked his tongue, and considered the tiles on the ceiling for a good four or five seconds. 'Are you familiar with the phrase, "done up like a kipper"?'

'I've heard it said on very old movies.'

'It's apt, in my case. Throughout my defence, led by the late, and most learned and esteemed Brian Vinnicombe QC, I was told that this should not be mentioned, and that her evidence would not be deemed admissible in court. He said that she would hinder my case, not help it.'

'But… she was your alibi, surely. How on earth could that not be relevant?'

'Oh, it wasn't irrelevant. The word I used was "inadmissible". You can ask her why, if they'll let you in. You'll probably have found it easier to speak to me in this place, rather than speak to her.'

'Why – is she in prison for something?'

'No, but she is locked up. Secure unit. Mentally ill.'

'What type of mental illness?'

Solomon scratched his beard. 'You know, nothing I could identify, looking back on it. I wouldn't have said she was ill, but she was twisted. We shared similar appetites, but she was way off the deep end.'

'Appetites? What do you mean by that?'

'Go ask her. A father shouldn't share that stuff with his daughter. That's just perverse!'

'Well, what happened to her?'

'She had cracked by the time I came to court, completely gaga. Not of this earth. She denied ever seeing me, ever knowing me. That was the only stuff that made sense.' He swallowed, and sat forward. Then something extraordinary happened; he put his head in his hands, and he sagged. Then he slapped himself, twice, as if returning to sensibility. She noted that his eyes were raw and red. 'We had something, Carol and I. I can't believe what happened, can't believe how quickly she went downhill… I've got my suspicions, you know.'

'About what?' She could barely believe his response, how quickly it came on. And yet he was genuinely crestfallen. It was the first time he had sounded remorseful. It was the type of tension release, that grief detonation, that could arrive suddenly. Freya knew all about that.

'It sounds paranoid. But God knows what pressure they put her under. For months on end. All the time I was on remand. Gnawing at her, knowing she would make me a free man… I have a lot of suspicions, put it that way. On top of that, I wouldn't be surprised if Brian Vinnicombe QC, God rest his soul, actually wanted me to end up in prison. You could say we didn't see eye to eye. Add these two elements together, on top of Bernie Galvin's shenanigans… Sorry, you want me to stop? You can catch your breath, if you like.' He indicated Freya's notepad; she was taking notes at quite some pace.

She took him up on his offer, making sure she wrote clearly and carefully, underlining certain parts. 'This is incredible… Thanks for this. I mean, it's extraordinary.'

'And I haven't even told you the best part. About these little whispers I heard. And the reason Bernie Galvin's lost the plot.'

'Go on.'

He winked. 'Oh, I have to keep back the odd secret. Where would be the fun in spilling my guts about everything? You'll find out soon enough.' He signalled to the guard; the interview was over.

20

The wooden fencing hemmed her in on either side, the alleyway constricting as before. Freya had a sudden flashback to the axe in the skull, and the chill damp of the unquiet grave she'd helped disturb. As the boarding scrolled past her, she imagined a worm, and its food passing through its guts.

She grit her teeth, and shook her head. She pushed on. Stay steady, stay strong, and push through.

When the graffiti appeared, it was so jarring she stopped completely, calves and thighs seizing up. Indigo blue spray paint, lettering a foot or more high, stretching along one side of the wall.

FREYA.

On the other side of the fence, there was smaller, denser text. She had to peer closely to read it.

After she'd taken a picture on her phone, she ran back out of the alley, utterly convinced someone was behind her, in front of her, running parallel on the other side of the fence. When she emerged into the main street, she cried out, wheezing, bent almost double.

She lifted her phone, made a decision, and called Glenn.

Freya checked there was no one around on the bus to overhear, then she whispered in Glenn's ear: 'It said, "The Mystery machinery moves slowly." Then it said: "The 49er knows where the Cyclops grows."'

'Right… That means nothing to me,' Glenn said.

'Mystery Machine is to do with Scooby-Doo. That's what Shaggy and Velma and the gang all travelled in – their psychedelic van.'

'This is a bit before my time.'

'You don't know Scooby-Doo? This is classical scholarship, here. There's a monster in Scooby-Doo called the Miner 49er. Old guy, beard, hat, up to some scheme or other down a mine. That got me thinking, after what you said…'

'And the Cyclops?'

'Not sure of the connection there. But I guess we're going to find out.'

Glenn ate crisps the way a squirrel might; his hands moved so fast you had to slow the film down a little to see them, and his jaws clashed in rapid-fire. 'I've got a hunch,' he said.

'Like the Hanging Oak?' Freya asked. They were sat on the top deck of a bus. It was a fine May morning, with blossom on the trees falling as the window brushed the trailing branches.

'Kind of. There was a bit of logic to that. But this is different. This is more of a hunch, and could turn out to be absolutely nothing. Sure you won't have a crisp?'

'…I still get spots.'

'I don't mind if you don't.'

Freya demurred. 'So, what's your hunch based on?'

'Well – you told me Mick Harvie gave you the tip-off about a ghost town. And then your dad told you something about a quarry. This seemed strange to me, as the Woodcutter case never focused on either of those things, so far as anyone knows.'

'It's from the police – so they're bound to keep some stuff back in their investigations.'

'Oh, that doesn't matter, after a while. I find out everything, eventually. Retired policemen sometimes get involved on the message boards, people who worked the cases. Journalists too. They want to get involved. Get the cases solved, you know? I've seen detailed transcripts of press conferences, had more than one source working on the case who confirmed details that Bernie Galvin gave at briefings… No sign of a quarry or a ghost town. But the two could be linked. So, I carried out a search for those, and…' He dug out his phone.

Freya narrowed her eyes at the image. 'I've no idea what that is. A cave? A stain on the wall? Something unspeakable?'

'The first answer was closest. That's an old slate mine. West Wales. St Mervyn's.'

'That'll be why we're going to Wales?'

'Yep. I've booked us a room, too. I hope you don't mind – you said you were free, the next couple of days.'

'Must have cost you. How much?'

'We can sort it out later. I can set up a bank transfer.'

'Nah, I don't do those. Cash is fine.'

Glenn arched an eyebrow. 'It's the twenty-first century,

you know. They have safeguards and what have you. Encryption.'

'And I just told you, I don't do bank transfers. I used to work in finance. In a phone farm. For a glorious three-week spell, I handled the complaints desk. That's the really, really persistent people who get past the automation. I've investigated their complaints. These things aren't as safe as you think.'

'OK.' He was bemused by this. 'I guess there's a bank machine at the station. Plus, you can buy me dinner.'

'Why do I feel as if I'm in a snare?' She grinned, and snatched at his crisps. By reflex his hand scrunched up the bag. Reluctantly, he unclenched his fist and the bag tried to return to its previous shape, like a ragged flower.

'Think I'll buy you cheese and onion for your dinner. Go exotic.'

'People will think we're a couple,' he said. Then he stared out the window, and it was hard to tell if he was blushing.

'Well, people can think, can't they?'

No one spoke for a moment or two, and they listened to the rumble and cadence of the bus. She had no idea why she'd said this… Or maybe she did. Maybe this was like Stuart Russell, her first and only crush from school. She could cringe at any time at the merest mention of his name. She'd bombarded him with calls, she'd written him notes in class, she'd even gone to his house, but Stuart Russell, all five feet six and fourteen years of him, had not been interested. It had taken a long time for her to recover from Stuart Russell – socially, she probably never did. Except the situation wasn't analogous. She didn't fancy Glenn, of course. But she needed him beside her. A partner, lower case p, rather than another half. Someone to share the load.

She studied the side of his face for a second or two, the hair straggling over his almost comically small ears. And what went on in Glenn's head? There was no doubt that in this scenario, Freya was the most important – and that might be the first time she could ever have said that about herself with any degree of confidence. So was Glenn only using her?

Guess we'll find out, sooner or later.

The road to the old slate mine was a different type of physical challenge to the ones Freya was used to. In her way she enjoyed the slower drag on her muscles, the fight against gravity, as opposed to the plodding monotony of a run. Glenn fared less well, but he lasted the pace. She took a quiet satisfaction in knowing she was fitter than him, but perhaps not by much.

'Perfect place to hide a car, if you were a killer,' he said, as they climbed a path made of broken slate.

'The road's wide enough, too. Used to be a working road – tarmac, the lot. It's broken up; grass and weeds did that, over time. You can still make the route out. Walkers' path, now.'

'Haven't seen any others out here, today.'

'No.' Glenn nodded towards a curve in the hills, which rose steeply on either side of them. 'I reckon I can see an entrance, there.'

'We're not going in it, surely? I was born to have adventure, but spelunking wasn't part of my diary today.'

'Nah. We're going to see if anyone's been in it recently. If the cops have found anything recently, it'll be taped off.' He stopped to take a drink of water, then consulted an OS map. Not too long ago it had been pristine, delivered after an online order just that morning. Already it was showing the scars of use in the field; untidy creases, and a little bit soggy in places. 'We're definitely on track.'

The mouth of the slate mine was indeed tightly fenced off, with the feel of a medieval trellis dropped across the entrance to a castle. Furthermore, police tape criss-crossed the entrance, warning people not to enter.

'That's that,' Freya said. 'Unless you really want to try and get in.'

'Nah. We've seen what we came for.'

'So that's it? That's what you dragged me out here for, really? To make sure the police had been here?'

'Yeah. It means what your dad and Mick Harvie say checks out, perfectly. But there's something else we need to look at.'

Freya placed a hand on the small of her back, and stretched, relieving some tension back there. 'The ghost town.'

'Right. St Mervyn's, they called it. Accommodation built for the miners. Not even so much of a town. Crappy little quads. Some of it burnt out, but it was too high up and too remote to bother with demolishing. Some folk use the units as bothies, but they've become unsafe. It doesn't even have a name on the maps, any more. I think the caves might have a clue of some kind for the police. But the ghost town will have a clue for us.'

'You mean like the Hanging Oak?' As soon as she said the

words, she had an unnerving flashback: the muddy yellow of bone left in the earth for a long time; the lacquered handle, still good enough to swing; and the dull metal lodged inside. Freya wanted to cover her eyes, blink it clear.

Perhaps Glenn had had a similar experience. He swallowed, then said: 'Yeah.'

'I'm thinking we might find another body here.'

'You might be right. Though we might find nothing. This could be a complete shot in the dark. We might have got nothing but blisters out of this. And don't forget, the police were here recently. You'd have thought they would have found something.'

'They were ham-fisted when it came to the investigation long ago. They might be equally clumsy now.' Freya glanced up at the sky. 'We should probably have stayed overnight and set out at first light. Time's getting on. How far away is the town?'

Glenn checked the map again. 'We don't head for the summit – we take the road around this mountain, leading away from the old pithead, then head down to the valley. St Mervyn's, or what's left of it, should be down the mountain in the valley.'

'And you brought your metal detector?'

He patted the backpack. 'Don't leave home without it.'

Freya shivered. 'There's one big question about all this. Something I don't get.'

Glenn looked tense. 'Go on.'

'Why? Why are we getting these clues? Why is this being exposed, now?'

'We talked about this before – the real killer wants us to find it, is my best guess. Or maybe your dad wants us to find the clues – maybe he thinks it'll help spring him. Those are the two logical answers, right?'

'I suppose… Part of me thinks he might be drawing us into the wilderness for a very bad reason.'

'We're almost there,' Glenn said, perhaps too keen to change the subject. 'We should still have some good light. I hope.'

21

It was overcast when they arrived at St Mervyn's, which didn't do much for its appearance.

How Freya had pictured the place wasn't too far away from the truth: two rows of cheap, brutalist cottage flats and bungalows, probably built in the early 1960s. They reminded Freya of an old secondary school she'd seen demolished in her home town, a couple of years before she had been due to attend it.

It seemed an obscenity that something so squat and functional should exist in lieu of such wonderful scenery; perverse that someone should have planned it that way. Nature had reclaimed a lot of the buildings, but nowhere near enough. Bushes had sprung out of broken roofs and guttering. Greenery was winning against the tarmac; the latter was in full retreat in the middle of the road, eruptions of grass and weeds corralling the grey and black into ever-decreasing segments. This pleased Freya's eye more than the broken windows and graffiti. A deer walking down the centre of the street would not have looked out of place, but a person would.

She said: 'Even if I was a rough 'n' ready wild-camping, backpackery-hillwalkery-type person, I wouldn't stay here.'

'Bit remote for your druggie set, but I get the point.' Glenn slid the OS map into a flap of his backpack. 'Timewise, we've probably got a couple of hours. We can always come back tomorrow morning if there's something we don't quite like the look of… Jesus.' His head jerked.

'What?'

'Thought I saw something move in one of the houses.'

'Where?'

'The last one on the left.'

Freya swallowed. 'I saw that movie.'

'Nothing there now. Or if it was, it's hiding.'

'Big or small?'

'I don't know,' he snapped. 'Not big enough to be a person.'

'You're sure?'

'Pretty sure, yes!' He stopped and stood up straight. She saw in his defensiveness that the tension had risen in him, just as the fear had swelled in her. Freya had a notion to take his hand.

Instead, she said: 'Sorry. I'm a bit keyed up. I shouldn't be so jumpy.'

'It's fine,' he mumbled, hitching up the backpack. 'Me too. I suppose. Best we get going. Something about this place.'

'I know what you're saying. Please don't say any more. Let's get in and get out.'

'Best we get looking. "Cyclops" is the key. Look for a house with one window. Something like that.'

Freya frowned. 'I hope it's more obvious. I don't fancy having to root through the cupboards and split floorboards in there.'

'I've had a look online... There doesn't seem to be anything that indicates a Cyclops or one eye or anything like that. Anyway, best we keep our eyes peeled. Or one eye, I should say.'

'Weather's about to turn crap,' Freya said, indicating a malevolent bank of grey cloud gathering overhead.

'Weather forecast told me it was going to be fine.'

'The sky's telling me it isn't. In fact...' Freya held out her hand, to catch the first heavy drops as they began to fall.

'Damn it.' Glenn shucked out a hood from a compartment at the back of his jacket. 'Best we pick up the pace, anyway. You'd think it was getting dark already.'

'I don't think we need to go too far,' Freya said, hunching as the rain came on more heavily.

'How's that?'

She pointed. 'Check it out.'

One of the buildings closest to the entrance to the street was shorter and blockier than the rest, with a full garden growing out of its roof. An ancient, pitted metal sign swayed slightly, at a right angle to the building; a pub sign, surely. Glenn squinted, but even from a distance Freya could make out the image on the front of the sign.

A giant, with what appeared to be a monk's tonsure, reaching out for tiny screaming matchstick men. A giant with one eye. 'The Blink And Miss It', was just about legible below.

'That's us,' Glenn whispered. 'In we go.'

As they drew closer, Freya made out a pair of pinwheeling legs angled out of the side of the giant's mouth. She felt a sudden sickness, and she stopped.

'Everything all right?' he whispered.

'We just take a look around,' Freya said, quieter still. 'Nothing daft. Agreed?'

'Course,' he said.

22

They used one of Glenn's shovels to pry open the chipboard that enclosed the front door. Immediately they were hit by a terrible smell; old books, soiled things, mould that would never be conquered.

Glenn cranked up a head torch, and fixed it around his head. Freya pulled out a heavy-duty torch, and soon the twin beams illuminated a musty, uneven wasteland. 'It's a real mess in there. And Jesus… Something moved.'

'Rats, surely,' Glenn said. 'Not a great fan of those.'

'After you, then.'

'Yeah. After me.'

Freya jerked back the board; it splintered in her hands, and she tossed the broken parts away. Glenn stepped through the gap. Something crunched under his feet.

'Was that glass?' Freya shone the torch onto the floor in the gloom of the pub. She could not quite dismiss the notion that the jagged aperture was a mouth, ready to seize her the moment she set foot over the threshold.

'Nah… Just old pallets, I think. No glass around here. No one's been squatting here for a while, and that's the truth. Just our four-legged friends, maybe.'

Freya stepped in alongside him. Their twin torch

beams criss-crossed through the darkness, illuminating a horseshoe-shaped bar. The light bounced off some cracked mirrors hanging around the back, but everything else had been stripped out. There were no taps, brasses or drinks gantries, no railings or jacket pegs. The top of the bar was garlanded with grime and dust, and some of the wooden panelling was scored with tiny claw marks.

'To be fair,' Freya said, 'I've been in pubs that looked worse.'

Glenn didn't laugh – but she saw a look of irritation cross his face. 'Maybe we should listen out, and maybe cut the jokes?'

'Sorry,' she whispered.

Maybe if I don't joke, Glenn, I'll scream.

Beneath some cracked shards of pallet, some chequerboard tiling was just about visible. Footprints were apparent in places, some bearing the heavy tread of hiking boots in thick brown islands, isthmuses and archipelagos.

'Those footprints – any of them look fresh to you?' he asked.

Freya shook her head. 'Hard to tell. What's the next part of the plan?'

'Well, I have a horrid idea that whatever we need to find in here is in the cellar.'

'Of course. The fucking cellar.' She regretted saying it; her voice quivered a little as she did so. *Scaredy cat.* She took one or two deep breaths, but they were not enough to still her heart. *Get away from this. This isn't like at the care home. Get out. Go home. This is not a place for you.*

She grit her teeth. *Rubbish. Get on with it.*

'Don't suppose you've got any heavy-duty tools in your

backpack? Getting into the cellar might be a problem otherwise.'

'Sure.' Glenn rooted around in the bag, and removed a sledgehammer. It looked as if it was from a different era in human history, its head rusted, its corners out of shape. Glenn let the head drop into the palm of his free hand with a smack; it still had some weight to it. Freya understood now why he'd been sweating so freely on the walk. 'I came prepared.'

Freya smiled, and reached into her own backpack, bracing the torch awkwardly under her chin as she did so. 'As did I.' She produced a crowbar, thick, black and with a wicked curve at the edge; a harpooner's instrument.

The weapons caught the bluish light; Freya felt a curious sense of impotence, now that she held the crowbar in her hands. She imagined having to smash it into someone – perhaps a moving target, a spindly figure creeping after them in the shadows.

Something shifted in a corner, out of the torchlight, and she came close to panicking then. The crowbar clattered to the floor; her torch beam scored crazed arcs and loops over the damn walls until Glenn's hand steadied her.

'Easy. It was a bird, flying out one of the broken panes.'

'Definitely?'

'For sure. I saw it.'

'OK.' She was not OK, though. Her heart was pounding, and sweat dripped down her chin. She heard herself say: 'I'm going to get this over with.'

Wincing, Freya vaulted onto the top of the bar, slid her legs over to the other side, and then lowered herself to the floor. For one awful moment, she couldn't see the floor beneath, and wondered if it had perhaps been eaten away, or collapsed into the cellar below. But she landed on old floorboards, which sprung slightly under her weight. She brought the torch down to focus on the grimy flooring. Brass edges delineated the cellar; there was a lock at the far edge.

'That's it,' she said.

'Dammit, that looks awkward,' Glenn said, his face obscured by the blue flare of light at the centre of his forehead. 'I was hoping for a padlock we could get through, easily enough.'

Freya held up the crowbar into the light. 'Here we go, then. Best to start with this.' She eased off her rucksack, then braced the crowbar in the gap between the edge of the trapdoor and the edge of its frame.

She gritted her teeth, took the strain, and heaved.

'Hey,' Glenn said, 'it's moving.'

With a brittle crack, something gave way under the crowbar, and the trapdoor opened. A quite awful smell appeared; Freya was reminded of an underpass her mother had warned her about in childhood, but which she dared herself to go down, anyway. It had smelled a bit like this: old beer, old piss, and sheer, throbbing malice.

All the way through her life, there had been no one to hold her hand. No one to put their hand to her back, when she was frightened. Her mother's love had been strong, but it had been smothering, in its way. She'd recognised that, but never shied away from it. So when Glenn's hand touched her back, briefly, she felt an absurd sense of gratitude.

'Nice work,' he said.

They stooped, both gaining a fingertip's width of grip around the gap. Glenn's face was very close to Freya's, fully lit by the torch she'd placed on the floor – so much that she could feel warmth radiating off him. 'On three,' he said. 'One, two…'

The hatch sprung open after some initial resistance. It leaned slightly to one side, and wouldn't quite remain upright. Freya was reminded uncomfortably of a shark's fin. 'Fair drop, down there,' she said, picking up the torch.

'Looks like there's some barrels.' Glenn shone his light off metallic edges.

'Any coffins?'

At this, something shrieked and burst out of the trapdoor.

Glenn screamed and sprang back. Freya was too shocked to move; finally her torch beam lit on a scuttling brown shadow, just in time to see its flapping worm tail whip the edge of the bar and disappear over the top.

'God almighty,' Glenn said, his breathing stertorous. 'God help us if someone is waiting for us down there.'

'Don't even think it. Surely not… It's been sealed, and it's dark.' She tried to banish some juvenile, but truly awful fantasies, then; images of silver-eyed vampires, of slavering demons.

Freya leaned over the edge, her torchlight reflecting off rows of sullen-looking beer barrels. Some looked modern, while some were wooden, like casks of whisky she'd seen on a distillery tour in Scotland her mother had taken her on when she was younger. Some had tarpaulin covering them, spectral figures in the gloom. Freya imagined children hidden underneath, stifling giggles.

'How'd the rat manage to get out of there, anyway?' Glenn said. 'And more importantly, how are we going to get down? That's quite a drop.'

'Over there.' Freya pointed, just inside the trapdoor, and to the left. 'There's a ladder. It's hidden among the old pump fittings. Hang on…' She reached across the gap, trying not to imagine a swarm of pointy-nosed, shrieking demons suddenly flooding over her hand and engulfing her. She used the hook of the crowbar to snag the end; it was on a pulley of some kind. With a grating sound, the ladder rolled across its fitting, before presenting itself to Freya.

'All the rungs and in place,' she said. 'Hold the torch, a minute.'

'You're going down now?'

'Yeah. Why else did we come here, if we're not going to have a proper look?'

'I didn't think we'd have to do a ladders 'n' levels kind of puzzle,' Glenn said, tetchily.

'We're coming down here to clear my father,' she said, her voice harsher than she'd intended. 'If it wasn't for that, you wouldn't get me within a mile of this place.'

'I didn't expect some kind of board game,' he muttered, a little hurt.

'Stands to reason that our tormentor wouldn't make it easy for us. If there's something hidden down here, then he would want it to stay that way, surely. It wouldn't be too easy to spot.'

'It also looks like a trap.' His head torch beam swung away, and he made eye contact. 'Doesn't it?'

'You stay up here. I'll go down.'

Glenn glanced around. 'I don't think I got the better deal, all told. Can't we both go down together?'

'Nope. We both go down there, and we both get trapped, that's senseless. But if the killer sneaks up on you, and sticks an axe in the back of your head, then at least I'll know he's around and I've got something to deal with.'

'Ten out of ten for pragmatism,' Glenn said, uneasily. 'I'll try to scream before I die, so that you get a warning.'

'Good lad. Right – here goes.' The first rung creaked, theatrically, but the ladder held strong. Freya tucked her torch into her pocket, and then lowered herself down into the pit.

23

Freya turned the torch onto the first cask. God knew what they would discover. She had to find out, but also didn't want to find out. This was the kind of dread and gloom and darkness that people tried to pretend didn't exist; she was flirting with the knowledge of an everyday thing that was best known by undertakers, care workers, the police, paramedics – things she'd known from her work in the care home, though never so gothic as this. The stuff of grim, ugly, grimy death.

Desiccated wisps of dead spiders added commas to the folds in the tarpaulin, knuckled legs bent over their heads. Freya pulled at the bluish material. Her nose was instantly tickled by the dust, and she sneezed.

'What's happening?' Glenn asked. She had moved out of the reach of his torch beam.

'Nothing. I'm having a look around.'

'Maybe see if you can break into one of the casks?'

'No, I want to check the place out first. If we're being guided towards something, they'll have left a sign.'

Underneath the tarpaulin was a large brandy barrel. It looked like it might have rolled off a merchant ship sometime in the early eighteenth century, perhaps somewhere with blue water and palm trees. She tested the wood with her finger; still solid, though the varnish had flaked away long ago, leaving burnished streaks.

She tested it with her shoulder; something sloshed inside. Keeping the beam fixed on the wood, Freya walked around the barrel. Then she gasped.

'Everything all right?' Glenn called.

'You should get down here,' she said, her throat dry.

'Hold on…' The ladder creaked; Glenn lowered himself down.

'Wait. Stay there,' Freya said. 'We shouldn't both be down here at the same time.'

'What is it, then? What can you see?'

Freya gripped the edges of the barrel and wheeled it round so that Glenn could pick it out with the torch beam. It was lighter than it appeared.

In the circle of bluish light, a single eye had been spray-painted.

'This is where we stop,' Glenn said. 'I say we call the cops. We're already in way over our heads, here. We should get in touch with the police, tell them what we know, and leave this the way we found it.'

'You're getting scared.' Freya nodded. 'I'm glad. I was worried you weren't getting scared. Because I'm absolutely bricking it. I am one hundred per cent getting scared.'

'I'm getting sensible. We could be messing with evidence, here. We contaminate something, the cops might think we put it there. But before we do…' He raised something that interfered with the steady beam of light.

'What are you doing?'

The click and whirr of his camera provided the answer. She hadn't even seen it in his hand. 'Already done,' he said, smugly, and disappeared back up the ladder.

Freya's torch beam danced over another tarpaulin-covered barrel. She noticed something spray-painted across this covering, the same colour of paint as the eye on another barrel. 'TWO WAYS', said the message.

'There's something here,' she said. 'Could be another message.'

The torchlight revealed something that looked like a trail of blood, poking out from underneath the tarpaulin – then she noticed that it was more spray paint: an arrow, heading into the filthy tarpaulin.

'Don't,' Glenn whispered.

But it was too late. She had already taken the tarp between her fingertips, lifted it, and there was the head of an axe, buried deep in the splintered barrel, the handle laid lengthwise across the top.

'Oh Christ,' she said, almost in a squeak.

'Be quiet,' Glenn hissed.

'You be bloody quiet!'

'There's someone out there!' His voice dropped to a whisper. Then the blue light from his head torch extinguished. 'Turn out your torchlight.'

'What do you mean?' Freya's heartbeat seemed to swell, soaking up all available space in the room. 'Can you see someone?'

'I can see them – there's someone walking around outside! Wait. Stay in there, and don't make a sound.'

'What? Don't you dare close that door!' she cried. But it

was too late. Glenn slid the trapdoor shut. Then she heard his footsteps creaking across the floor overhead, towards the front door.

Trying to control her breathing, she clicked off the torch beam, and waited.

There was silence from above. Then a sudden, grinding crash as something struck the panelling they had crept through at the front door. Then another. Then another. With every impact, Freya's shoulders cinched up tight. Her free hand flew to her mouth. There was no mistaking what this cacophony represented.

It was the sound of wood being chopped.

24

With a final crash, something heavy fell to the floor above. The board at the front entrance – no doubt about it.

Freya pinned herself against the far wall. Though it felt stuffy and dusty down there, the concrete at her back was cool. Sweat nonetheless began to form at her forehead, and tickle the base of her spine.

Footsteps, now, across the floor. Heavy boots, lumpen steps, almost as percussively brutal as the axe blows. And then something else; a heavy scraping or scoring sound.

Freya could picture the blade of the axe, dragging across the floor. Perhaps it left tiny shavings in its wake, a splintered slalom traced across the grain.

The footsteps were directly overhead. Whoever had come into the room had stopped at the bar.

The person up above tapped their feet once, twice, three times. Then they began to move around the bar, heading towards the trapdoor.

Freya darted forward, using the footsteps as cover for her own. She stopped at the ladder; placed her foot on the bottom rung, then boosted herself up.

She had spotted it on her way down – there was a catch,

which she had broken when she'd used the crowbar to jemmy open the trapdoor. Like an unbuckled belt, two parts of the latch hung downwards – it was where the padlock had hung in place, above.

She placed the crowbar in between these two bent pieces of metal, closing the two halves of the latch. At that precise moment, the trapdoor jerked.

The latch held; the crowbar clanked. Freya stepped back a moment. There was a sudden silence, then a clearly audible, 'Hmm.'

Then a terrible blow struck the trapdoor. The end of the crowbar jerked and dangled like a landed fish. Wood splintered, and a thin grey line appeared above Freya's head, as the entire trapdoor buckled.

Another blow staved it in even further. Freya saw a heavy black boot shifting; then a third crash brought the blade through the wood. Splinters cascaded down the ladder.

Utterly unnerved, Freya reached for the crowbar, yanking it free. Then she fled, crouching behind one of the barrels.

The figure above grunted. Then with a fourth terrific blow, the trapdoor split down the middle. A foot crashed down and sent both halves into the cellar.

Freya couldn't see who was up there. She heard heavy breathing – it was a man, surely, and one who'd exerted himself.

'Well now,' said a deep, gravelly voice. It was like someone snoring; the type that carried through walls from neighbours. 'Who have we got down there, then?'

Freya said nothing, clutching the torch with one hand, and the crowbar in the other.

'Whoever's down there, come out.'

He stopped moving; stopped breathing, perhaps. There was an awful silence. Surely he could hear her very heartbeat. She clamped a hand over her nose and mouth.

'I won't hurt you.'

The voice was familiar. But from where?

Freya closed her eyes for a second, visualising the layout of the pub above. She tried to remember if there'd been a grille or metal hatchway outside; she couldn't be sure if she'd imagined it, but was it to the left of the window?

She took a chance, and ran over.

There was a set of stairs there – metal, chrome-brushed, totally different to the stairs that led back to the bar. Freya clicked on her torch, having already broken cover. There, dangling from a similar latch to the trapdoor, was an old rusted padlock.

Perfect.

She made precise contact with the crowbar, hooking the padlock, and then snapping it with one wrench of her shoulders.

The intruder clattered down the rest of the steps. Running, now. 'Ahh, no you don't, no you don't...'

Freya was at the top of the steps in an instant, barging her shoulder into the twin doors above her head. She rebounded with a thick, gonging sound.

Directly ahead; a snib lock. She threw it, then got her shoulder against the hatch again, and then she was out into the sudden night.

'Wait!'

Freya did not wait. She hurled the twin doors back on the advancing figure, too dark to see any details.

Then she was sprinting down the crooked old street, as the hatchway outside grated open behind her.

On impulse she dodged down the side of one of the bungalows. Sprinting past a broken bathroom window with a mildewed shower curtain flapping around inside, she rounded a corner, fully intending to double back on herself.

That's when a hand reached out and grabbed her.

25

She shrieked – then gripped the figure by the throat, and drew back the crowbar.

'Freya! It's me, for God's sake!'

Glenn; Glenn's shocked face. His upper incisors poked out from beneath his top lip, and Freya saw herself releasing, shattering them, then following through—

'It's Glenn!' His other hand grabbed her wrist. She blinked, then lowered the crowbar. Her shoulders sagged. *Thank God.*

'He's there,' Freya whispered. 'Right behind me. We've got to think, think…' She screwed her eyes shut, and tried to visualise the layout of the cabins. 'One of those buildings just opposite is open. It's not obvious but there's a back door. It looks bolted shut, but it's open. We can lie low in there.'

'No… There's two of us. You've still got your backpack, the shovel. This is a chance to take him down.'

Freya shook her head. 'No way. This is a *multiple fucking murderer*. He's been in this situation before. No one's ever escaped from him. We're asking for it. I say we hide.'

'What, we hide until he gets the drop on us? There are two of us. We work together.'

'No,' she said, turning away. 'There's just one of you. You come with me, or you're on your own. This isn't sensible.'

Glenn grit his teeth, then followed after her. 'Come back here. We can take him down. We can actually catch him.'

'It's not on; it's not pragmatic. He'll kill us! This isn't a game. Come on!'

Still protesting, Glenn followed her around the corner, hugging the back of the buildings. Rudiments of old gardens were apparent here, placed where fences had once stood. Underneath, ancient flagstones and patios were choked and dismembered by weeds. Overhead, the daylight had all but disappeared, and much of what remained had been soaked up by clouds the colour of tombstones.

'In here, then, if we're hiding,' Glenn said, almost too low to hear. He indicated a dark door. Freya had an instinctive sense of repulsion to that gloomy portal. But she followed him.

There was hardly any light in the hallway; the floorboards creaked, Hammer Horror-movie style, and they both froze. 'Come on,' he whispered. They trooped into what must have been someone's front room. In the faint light Freya could make out a pile of wooden panels and brass fittings, as if a bed had simply flown apart in despair. Dark, jagged smears streaked the length of the far wall, surely of dark provenance. Bizarrely, a TV set was in the corner, a big-ticket purchase from about forty years ago, blocky and wood-panelled. The screen had been completely destroyed, not even baby-teeth shards remaining, with the space inside floored with straw. The place had a near-unbearable animal stink.

'Under the windowsill,' he said. The window was broad and fully intact, though coated with an accumulated patina of grime. Someone had run a finger across this substance, but only once, and not for long. The grime admitted only a thin grey light, smudging the far wall, illuminating a white circle where a wall clock had once ticked.

They both huddled down. The sill was broad, and anyone passing by would not be able to see who was in there.

'He might search the whole place,' Freya said. As quietly as she dared – and still too loud.

'He won't,' Glenn replied. 'It's a waste of time. We've found a body – this isn't safe for him.'

'What's he playing at? Why's he letting everyone know where the bodies are, after all this time?'

'Vanity? Messing with people? Who knows what's going on in his head? Maybe he's got a bigger plan. Maybe he's coming out of retirement.'

'This has got to prove, beyond a doubt, that my dad isn't the Woodcutter.'

'That's an assumption.'

Freya gripped Glenn's arm. 'Quiet…'

They sat on their haunches, listening to the creak and whistle of the wind through the house. The door rattled in a stiff breeze; a steady drip beat out its rhythm in the floor above.

Then they heard the footsteps outside.

It was a steady gait, utterly unconcerned about making a noise, on the pavement. Freya shrank against the peeling wallpaper. Her senses had been invaded not just by the smell of damp, but by the sense of it – everywhere. She covered her nose and mouth with her hands. She wanted to say it, again and again, a prayer or an incantation: *I don't want to be here. I don't want to be here…*

On the far wall, the smudge of light changed. A clear, thin shadow appeared. Then it became more distinct, and the footsteps came closer.

He was coming towards the window.

Freya let one hand drop down to the crowbar at her side. Her eyes met Glenn's for a moment. They were like hers; wide open, scared.

The window frame rattled once – not a blow, just someone testing the frame for any give. Not much was apparent. Then there was a moment of complete and utter silence, presided over by that terrible, thin shadow.

Then it slowly withdrew, and the footsteps receded.

Glenn reached for his backpack, but Freya shook her head, tapping her ear. They both listened to the footsteps recede. Then Freya pointed to her watch. *Two minutes*, she mouthed.

Once it had elapsed, Freya scuttled across to the far side of the room, still clinging close to the wall housing the window frame. 'I think that's it. He's gone.'

'I wouldn't be sure,' Glenn said. He dared a look over his shoulder, as he fit his arms into the backpack. 'Can't see anyone.'

'All clear from here. Get on over.'

'I can't be sure. He might be able to see you from an angle, over there.'

'Look, Glenn, I'll explain to you how light works another time. I can't see him. He's gone. Anyway, I don't think he wants to kill us. What's the point?'

'Yeah. No point giving us bodies to find, and then offing us.' Glenn began to crawl commando-style towards Freya. His backpack bobbed on his back, the world's most awkward armadillo. 'Maybe he's just trying to size us up, find out what he's dealing with. And scare us.'

The window erupted. Shards of glass exploded into the room; the entire pane disintegrated.

Freya covered her head, and screamed. Glenn rolled across the floor, scrambling for his pack. The shovel slithered out of his hands, and clanged on the floor.

Torchlight flooded the room, a keen, pale blue laser light that dazzled Glenn.

'For God's sake,' a voice said, almost on a chuckle. 'What are you *doing* in there?'

26

He kept them waiting out by his car. He did not invite them in, even when the rain began to fall heavier. Freya and Glenn kept their jackets zipped and their hoods tight over their heads. He kept a good distance from them, leaning against the side of his car. Freya realised she wanted to raise her hands; it was as if he held a gun on them.

DI Connor Tamm didn't bother with waterproofs, though he had a three-quarter-length wax jacket, walking trousers and heavy boots. Neither of these things looked as stained as they should have, while Freya and Glenn were daubed and pooled with mud in just about every angle of their joints.

Tamm's hair flitted about his head as the wind blew. 'One of these days, Freya, we'll meet somewhere where it's warm and dry. In fact, I think that day is going to be tomorrow.'

Freya had to speak up over the wind. 'Did you drive up here with the lights off? Weird that we didn't hear you drive in.'

'You must have been busy over at the ghost town. Yeah, I drove up here. I had to keep the lights on, though. You kidding? I don't want to end up over a cliff.'

'Just happened to be passing the area?' Glenn said, sourly.

Tamm grinned. He had an easy posture on the car, his hands linked over his flat stomach. 'I happened to be following you two. Call it a hunch.'

'I call it stalking.'

'This is a very serious investigation, Glenn,' Tamm said. 'It's not a joke. Our department – and God knows I keep complaining about this – doesn't have the money to carry out massive investigations. I'm doing the work on my own time. My wife is absolutely thrilled, I can tell you.'

'We came by train,' Freya said. 'How did you know we'd be here?'

'It's easy to keep track of train ticket bookings, when you're a policeman,' Tamm said.

'Remind me never to stiff a copper on eBay,' Glenn muttered.

Eager to draw Tamm's attention from Glenn's arch tone, Freya said: 'I'm assuming it was you, following us over the old pub.'

'It was me, all right. You had me spooked, I had to admit. I wasn't quite sure what I was going to find in there.'

'What did you find?' she asked.

'You tell me. I haven't looked inside the drum. I've an idea it might be something unpleasant. And I can tell you that when we checked this site a few weeks ago, there was no sign of any drum. And no weird writing on the walls, either.'

Freya and Glenn stayed silent.

Tamm leaned forward a little, and said, conspiratorially: 'Now. That's something off-the-record, me to you. How about you give me something in return?'

'We've nothing to give you,' Glenn said.

'Then you can answer my questions. How is it that a couple of days after I speak to you…' he pointed at Glenn; Freya realised for the first time that he was wearing gloves '…about finding human remains in the middle of a field, in the middle of nowhere, that you're in contact with the girl at the centre of the entire business, and then you arrive here, and find… what could well be another body? With another axe?'

Freya and Glenn studiously avoided each other's eyes. Freya said: 'We had an anonymous tip-off.'

Glenn tutted. Tamm glared at him for a second, but he said, in a kind tone: 'Can you explain a little bit more about that, Freya?'

She took a deep breath, and told him about the graffiti in the alleyway on her running route. 'I don't know where it came from. I got a tip to come out here…'

'Was this by phone?'

'I didn't say it was by phone,' Freya stammered.

'Yeah, and if it was by phone, you'd know that already,' Glenn sneered. 'Policemen have ways of tracking phone calls.'

Tamm ignored him. 'Freya,' the detective said, 'this isn't a courtroom drama on American television. If you know something and it's related to a crime, you have to report it to me.'

'That's all I want to say,' Freya said. 'It pointed to this area, so we came out.'

'How did you know to come to the pub?'

'We didn't,' Glenn said. 'We searched a few places. The pub was the most obvious building to go to.'

'I wasn't asking you,' Tamm said. 'Now, this tip-off…

Did it mention that the police had been here recently to carry out a search?'

'I don't want to say anything about that,' Freya said.

'So let's assume they did. That is interesting.' Tamm scratched his chin. 'We kept it very secret. All that search business. A former officer told us that he'd always had an inkling that there was a body hidden up here. Came from an eyewitness account of a black van being seen in the area, not long after Coleen Arden vanished. He never quite followed it up, he said. He'd been going over his notes, and found a reference. This tip-off – it didn't come from one of your acquaintances in the press, did it?'

Freya said nothing.

'Well. Never mind. I'll ask these questions again, but in a more formal setting. I can promise you one thing, though. A nice cup of tea.'

Tamm nodded to a point over Freya's shoulder. She turned around, in time to see the blue lights scoring pale strobing trenches along the winding road to the old mine.

27

Tamm's sidekick's name was Detective Sergeant Hunter, and he looked like a convict, rather than a policeman. His thumb-like features were squashed flat, with stubble on his head and chin the only thing delineating any features. He said very little in the interview room. Tamm said enough for both of them.

The detective inspector never became adversarial, but his tone wasn't quite as warm as Freya remembered. 'So you don't have any idea of your source? All you got was a piece of graffiti?'

'All of this was complete speculation.' Freya had gone beyond fear, now, somewhat reassured by Tamm's presence. 'We just put two and two together and, it looks like we got four.'

'One more time… What day did you get the tip-off?'

'It was the other day. Wednesday. I was going through one of my running routes…'

Tamm took up his pen, and fixed his notepad underneath his finger. 'Be specific. What route?'

'It's off Marley Street, a row of nice new houses – four and five apartments, red brick, detached. Fancy cars in the drive. There's an alleyway, connecting two estates. Quite narrow.

There's some boarded fencing on either side.' None of this was a lie, of course. Tamm would know, she supposed, if she did lie. 'My name was written on the boarding. Then it had the cryptic message, just as I said.'

'And if I was to send someone down there now, it'd still be there?'

'It's surely been removed now. But sure – have a look.'

Tamm leaned back in his seat. 'I would put it to you that it's quite odd that you didn't think to share this with us.'

'For all I know it was a crank. I have been in the papers. I've drawn attention to myself. That doesn't excuse anyone taking liberties, but it's a fact of life that it can happen.'

'You reckon you've got a stalker?'

'I reckon that the person who left the graffiti is the actual Woodcutter,' Freya said, carefully.

'And he may be stalking me, yes. But he's also sending me a message.'

'He's also sending the location of bodies to you.'

'Then there's a body in the barrel?'

Tamm nodded.

DS Hunter folded his arms, and chewed the inside of his mouth. Then he tutted, and said: 'I'd have an alternative theory, Freya. I'd say, it's possible that you left the graffiti yourself.'

'What?'

'It's just a theory, as I say. I'd suggest, you left the graffiti yourself. You hook up with Glenn Allander, and together you go to the old slate mine and the ghost town, and you somehow find the body in there. A body, in a place where the police had combed over just a few weeks before. So you make it look like someone's given you the information, but really, you had it all along. I'd also suggest that maybe you were Glenn's original source, when he somehow found this clue that took him to the Hanging Oak, and the first body. This is because you've been in contact with the only man ever convicted of being the Woodcutter – your father. It's awfully convenient that all this has come out after you found out he was your father, and then visited him in prison. Isn't it?'

Freya's eyes brimmed with tears, and her cheeks burned. She was embarrassed about letting her anger escape, but something about Hunter's demeanour demanded it. 'That's a load of bollocks – and you know it. How could my father have told me where to find bodies without anyone in the prison service or elsewhere knowing it? This is nonsense. I'm telling you the truth. What you believe is up to you.'

'I believe your father is the Woodcutter,' Hunter said. 'And he's feeding you information.'

'You can believe what you like.' She looked towards Tamm. *No... Don't do that. Looking for reassurance, help or shelter from the big kind doggie? This is exactly what they want. They're playing a game, and you're going along with it.*

'We'll check all this out,' Tamm said. 'I think you'd agree that it is extraordinary that you should get two pieces of information on the location of bodies that we've been trying to find as long as you've been alive.'

'What was the second piece of information?' Freya asked.

A slight smile from Tamm. 'I'm including Glenn Allander finding the first body.'

'Sure.' *He must have found the arrows in the forest, surely*. 'Right after he met me... But not before.' *He must have been blind not to see them. Police notice things – that's their job.*

Tamm leaned forward and linked his hands together on the desk, 'I'm going to ask you really nicely, Freya, because I'd hate you to get into any trouble. If you get any tips, any steers at all, from anyone, get in touch. Concealing knowledge of a crime is in itself a crime. I don't say that to scare you.' His kind smile came out, for the first time. 'Or maybe I am.'

'I'll bear it in mind.'

Freya didn't like DS Hunter's answering grin.

Once they met up again, underneath the painful white light outside the police station, Freya said: 'Pint?'

'Oh yeah,' Glenn said. 'Pint. For sure.'

They found a chain pub that seemed absurdly busy, until they saw the two-for-one promo blackboard. Thankfully there was a high table with awkward stools, close to the bar. Freya told herself she'd have one drink, and make it last. Glenn matched her sip for sip, carefully.

'It must look as if we're up to something,' Glenn said. 'They kept coming back to how I got the first tip-off. They know I'm talking nonsense.'

'We are up to something.' Freya took a quick sip, scanning the faces queued up at the bar over Glenn's shoulder. A mixed bag of ages; possibly even an office night out, judging by the collar and ties. Maybe even a police department night out. 'You're right, though. We'll need a more convincing cover story than the ones we've put together so far.'

'Probably watching us,' he muttered.

'Possibly watching us. Tamm was keen to tell me how little money and resources they've got to follow people. They have to do it on their own time. Imagine that. If they are, they'll struggle to know what we're up to. If we are up to anything.'

On a sudden impulse, she pushed her stool over beside Glenn, then sat down, her hip nudging his. He seemed panicked by this, lurching back alarmingly.

'You've got sauce on the side of your mouth,' Freya said, leaning in close. 'No... the other side.'

Glenn surveyed the red smear on his napkin. She laid a hand on his shoulder, and leaned in closer. 'Can a chicken look startled?' she asked him.

'Eh? How do you mean?'

'Because if it can, that's what you look like, right now.' Her lips were close enough to brush his earlobe.

'What's this?' he whispered.

'I don't want to get any on me.'

'Any what?'

'Ketchup. Look, here's how it goes. For any witnesses or CCTV cameras who might take an interest – we're going to look like a couple on a dirty weekend.'

Freya took his hand. For a second, he froze. Then he drew his thumb across the back of her hand, gently.

She smiled. 'That's it. You're getting the idea. Incidentally, back at the ghost town... Thanks for stepping in. I mean, for all you know, there was a maniac after me. You thought fast.'

'It might still be a maniac. Face it. Tamm could be the Woodcutter. He's older than he looks. And you said something about how they reckon it's a big coincidence that you've shown up just as the bodies start appearing. I reckon it's an even bigger coincidence that Tamm has popped up all of a sudden just as we get these tip-offs.'

'I don't think Tamm's got anything to do with it. But I'll keep an open mind. Thanks, anyway. For shutting me in in the dark, with a corpse. That's your take-home message. You're a bit of a hero.'

'All I could think to do,' he said. 'He was coming over at some pace. I didn't think you had a chance to get out in time. He would have caught you.'

'He would have caught me anyway if I hadn't gotten out of the outside cellar door, but we'll leave that aside.'

Glenn was looking at her lips, openly, now. He continued to stroke the back of her hand. Then his fingers interlocked with hers. It tingled. 'I suppose I came good in the end.'

'Are you actually flirting with me?' She spluttered laughter.

'I don't know. Maybe. Maybe we should look like a couple. Throw any watchers off the scent.'

'If we look like a couple, it would look like we were definitely up to something.' The excitement throbbing in her veins was out of control; she might twitch – her feet might leave the ground. It had been a while since anything like this had happened. Too long.

'Maybe we are up to something.' His gaze went to her mouth.

'Maybe I should kiss you, then.'

He swallowed. She noticed his lips quaked as he spoke. 'Maybe you should.'

She did kiss him then. Very briefly. He licked his lips when she drew back – a nervous gesture. His leg was quivering under the table; she wanted to burst out laughing at this.

'People have to see us doing this, yeah?' he said.

'Yeah. We should make a real show of it.' And she took him in her arms.

28

They had coffee together at the station café, after taking the train back to the city. They didn't hold hands, but he rested his shin against hers under the table. They talked about murder, of course.

'This all suggests he's a trophy hunter,' Glenn said. 'I always assumed the bodies had been buried somewhere very remote or very clever, where it'd take a massive fluke to find them.'

'I'm not sure about that,' said Freya. 'For my money, he's all over the place. The MO is slippery. In the last case, June Caton-Bell, the one they fitted up my dad for – the body was left for people to find. Or, what was left of it, anyway. Keeping a body in a barrel seems a radical change.' She shivered, squeezing her eyes shut. She remembered the raw reek of the barrel – alcohol, possibly formaldehyde. She had an image of a body suspended in a sunless sea, dark hair streaming out behind it, obscuring the face, arms outstretched.

A warm hand closed over hers. 'You going to be all right, Freya?'

'Yeah. Sure. Why not?'

'Because a lot of things have happened to you in a very

short space of time. You're going to crash, at some point. Take it from me.'

'I'll be fine.' She smiled, none too convincingly. 'You know, when I worked in the care home… I saw death, quite a lot. Sometimes it was dignified, but just as often, it wasn't. I remember Mrs McAneney. She died on the throne. She had a brilliant sense of humour; I could imagine her laughing about it. But when I heard one of the older hands making a joke about her… I didn't lose my temper. But I knew I had to leave. That was bad enough. But this kind of death, this guy… It's a different world.'

'Not your world, Freya. Whatever we see, we have to hold on to that.'

Freya missed Glenn's touch, when she withdrew her hand. She shook her head. 'I'm fine. I'll keep going. You must admit… in a way, it's exciting, all this. And we have to focus on the goal. It'll help get my dad in the clear.'

'That something you really want?'

'Course it is,' Freya said, sharply. 'Why wouldn't I? You said it yourself – he's innocent.'

'I think the person leaving us the clues is *probably* the Woodcutter – it stands to reason. That's probably, in italics. I didn't say your dad was innocent. And as you say – there's a big difference in the way the bodies were found in June Caton-Bell's and Max Dilworth's cases. Out of the three bodies we've got so far, Dilworth and this second body were placed there for you to find. Not as gory or shocking as a pile of body parts, but theatrical enough. So, it could be that your dad killed June Caton-Bell. That's a well-known theory in the case – that he was guilty of chopping up June Caton-Bell and making it look like the Woodcutter's work.

But he wasn't the actual Woodcutter, who murdered the rest.'

'I've done my research, too,' Freya said. 'Plus I've read the same reports you have, on the tests they've done with Max Dilworth's remains.'

Glenn frowned. 'How did you get those? Your newspaper guy?'

Freya dismissed the question. 'My point is, it seems Dilworth and Caton-Bell were chopped by the same person. A lot of similarity in the cuts, in the killing rage. The overkill. Seems the axeman's stance was exactly the same, in those cases. That'd disprove your theory.'

'They're only theories. But at the moment, I'd say your mystery man is the top candidate. And he's getting awfully agitated. Or at least, awfully busy.'

'What's the point of that, though? To stay quiet all these years, then start getting active again?'

'It's not uncommon. The Green River Killer, and one you might not know, called BTK – Bind, Torture, Kill. Both had major hiatuses in cases, because they got married. Steady relationships calmed them down, for whatever reason. Maybe it gave them an outlet for their urges that didn't involve killing. Maybe it gave them love and support they'd never had before. Or maybe it just made them feel normal. But they both came back for a late crack at it. BTK was traced through email metadata, of all things. He tried to taunt the police after he came out of retirement. That's how they got him. Because he was an email noob.

'So, maybe there's been a major change in our guy's life. Or maybe he was just triggered by all the attention of late. It can't be easy, being someone in that position. If you think about it. He'll maybe want the acclaim and glamour of being a famous murderer. The fact that he frightens people. The fact that he got away with it. But he's also a pragmatist. So, along comes a golden chance. Someone to take the blame for him. So, he takes it, and he lies low.

'But then he starts getting annoyed. Part of the juice for being a killer is the idea that you're getting away with it – that every police officer in this part of the land is looking for you, that people will write books or newspaper features about you. And then up pops your dad – taking the blame, but also taking the credit for your work. Maybe, seeing his daughter so prominently in the papers was the real spur. Maybe he wants the credit, now? Maybe he doesn't like your dad getting the praise for the work he didn't do?'

Freya shrugged. 'Intriguing stuff, all the same. So – next step?'

Glenn paused. 'You mean the Woodcutter, or… us?'

'Stick to the Woodcutter for now. We've got plenty of time for an "us".'

Glenn beamed. 'Well. Right. That's… that's a good thing. Isn't it?'

'Course it is.'

'OK. I'm glad. Now about the Woodcutter… I think we wait to see if there's an official announcement from the police, saying they've found a third body. They've got a lot of forensics to get through before any formal announcement is made. Probably we should wait until then. Or, we have a race – I'll lean on my sources, you lean on yours, and the winner calls up first?'

'Deal.' They shook on it.

At that moment, Freya's phone buzzed; a text message. It seemed to throb on her screen.

'I've got him.'

29

It was from Mick Harvie.

Freya waited until she'd said goodbye to Glenn and caught the bus to her flat before answering the text, trying not to show her agitation, or plain excitement. *I wonder how many tells I dropped there?* she wondered, waving goodbye out the window.

She texted back: 'Got who? The Woodcutter?'

He called her immediately, startling her. Freya made sure that Glenn had disappeared from view before clicking on the blinking screen.

'The Woodcutter?' Harvie chuckled. 'No, they've got the Woodcutter already. I told you that.'

'Don't keep me in suspense then, Mick. Who have you got?'

'Bernard Galvin. You remember? The ex-copper. The man who was in charge of the Woodcutter inquiry. He's been in and out of the new headquarters in Leeds more times than some coppers who still actually work there. Very agitated old boy, is Bernie, according to my old snitches. And I find that very interesting.'

'So – what, is he here with you now?'

'Nah, I've managed to track him down. He had gone

to ground. Seems the old investigation is getting too hot. That body you turned up at the farmer's field was a little bit awkward for everyone. Especially with your dad's appeal coming to a close. I got a very polite brush-off from the plod, every time I asked to speak to him. He won't answer his phone, apparently.'

'Where is he, then?'

'If you want to know where he is, you'll have to come along with me to speak to him.'

'What's that going to turn up? He can slam a door in my face just as easily as yours.'

'I think he's less likely to close the door on you. You're *interesting*, love. To the police, and to people like me. You've put yourself out there – and now you're linked to a body.'

'So, let's say I speak to him… What's the point?'

'It'd be an exclusive for you. Anything he says to the Woodcutter's daughter is going to be news. If I tell you where he is, you can approach him, and we can half in for the fee.'

'How about I find him myself and tell you to get stuffed?'

'You'll never find him.' Harvie's tone was infuriatingly jolly – that of a mid-tier school bully with something to sneer about. 'Talk sense. I've got the goods, and I've got the contacts. You, however, are an angle. Mix it all together, and it's the perfect recipe.'

'How did you find him?'

'I'm not part of the dark side, as such, but I know a guy who knows a guy who happened to owe me a little favour. He told me where Bernie's hiding out. Strange that he should head all the way out there. Not like him. The Bernie Galvin I knew liked to lead from the front. Big face, thick neck, big voice. Hiding isn't his thing. He's not under police protection, either.'

'Maybe he thinks the real Woodcutter's still out there?' Freya asked. 'Maybe he thinks the Woodcutter's going to find him?'

'Nah, I told you – your dad's the Woodcutter. Believe it. But I've heard that there's a lot of activity in the old case. The kind that might get your dad out of jail. So that's kind of why I want you to knock on Galvin's door. I'll provide the rest of the cover – pictures, and such. All you have to do is try to find out what the score is with the Woodcutter inquiry. Has it been fully reactivated? What's Bernie's role? Has he been brought in as a consultant? That kind of thing.'

'It's tempting.'

'And of course, there's money in it for you.'

'I'm not doing this for money.'

'Course you aren't.' He might as well have hissed this. 'Nonetheless, I'll mention a figure. We'll see if you agree.'

He told her. She gave an ironic, stage whistle. 'Is that just half of it, or the full amount?'

'That's just your half. If we deliver for the paper.'

'What am I supposed to "deliver", exactly?'

'A few words, that's all. Ask him about Max Dilworth. Ask him about your dad. Spook him. Or... charm him. Bernie Galvin had an eye for the young ones.'

'I'm not so young,' Freya said, sullenly.

She held her ear away from the sudden, rasping laugh. 'Oh yes you are! So – do the numbers sound good? Are you in?'

'When do you want to do this?'

'Today sound all right? I don't want him to get restless and move on somewhere without us. If I've found out about it, one or two others might have.'

'OK. It'll take me a while. I'm travelling by train. What's the nearest station to where Bernie Galvin is?'

Harvie tutted. 'Hmm. That would be telling. Why don't I come and meet you wherever you are, and drive you?'

'No thanks.'

'It's no trouble.'

'I'm sure it isn't. I just don't trust you. Tell me the nearest train station, and you can meet me there.'

Harvie sighed. Then there was a long silence. Freya checked her screen to make sure the call was still connected. Finally, he said: 'All right then. I can tell you where he is. Do you fancy a day at the seaside?'

She sent Glenn a text. 'Had to go back. Sorry. Things to go through at Mum's. Will sort out my half of the hotel bill.' Then, hurriedly, after she'd sent that one: 'Enjoyed my night very much. Catch up soon. Pints in a coupla days?'

While she waited at the bus stop for a connection, Glenn tried to call. This being ignored, he sent her a single text: '…Er, also the matter of debrief? We need to talk things through. How about Carol Ramirez?'

'Aw, Glenn,' she whispered, as the bus pulled up. She didn't want to involve him this closely in whatever Mick Harvie had to offer. There was a sense of betrayal; but also, she didn't want to pull Glenn into Harvie's orbit.

Or maybe you're still a little bit competitive over your dad. You don't want Glenn getting the full story. And you aren't quite ready to share your dad with him that much. Isn't that the truth?

Perhaps this inner voice was like her mother's. At any rate, maybe it spoke an uncomfortable truth.

She sent Glenn one last text: 'Sorry. More soon. Got to go. Don't mean to seem weird.'

The run through to the seaside was a tonic for Freya. There was a break in the weather, and the dull clouds that had settled over the mountains gave way to patches of brilliant blue. Despite a long night in more than one manner of speaking and a stressful day, she felt her spirits lift along with the gulls.

When she was younger, Freya had imagined becoming rich, possibly famous, or maybe simply solvent. Mary had been prudent, but never flashy; she'd had plenty saved, thank God, to allow Freya a degree of comfort for the time being. But Freya had always thought of a day when she might take her mother out for a drive – maybe a bit of shopping, maybe a fancy lunch. The fantasy had grown into a day in a convertible car. The top would be down, and their hair would be flying. Now that was an impossibility, she transferred this to the possibility that she might have a similar day with her father. This was absurd for a lot of reasons, but she didn't deny herself the sense of comfort, the idea of a day at the seaside, walking down the prom, getting an ice cream or a bag of chips, skimming stones into the sea. The idea of a comforting hand at her back, again.

The train sliced through the valleys towards the coast. Endearingly, before the train reached the end of the line, some of the stations were request-only stops. She had never encountered these before. *Perhaps the diesel will morph into a steam train before I get off*, she thought. She imagined a leering, demonic face on the front of such an engine, before she could stop herself. Even so, she considered having a drink by the time she got off at the terminus.

She had had one and was considering another when Mick Harvie showed up. He had on a green military-style jacket with packed pockets, over the top of a black polo shirt, all of which suited his wiry frame. Freya noticed he'd trimmed his beard, too. She wouldn't have gone so far as to call him handsome, but he was at least presentable. When he came forward to shake her hand, she smelled a pungent aftershave, and then knew for certain that he'd dressed up for her.

'Can't believe you beat me to the station,' he said, sardonically. 'I had a few roadworks on the way, but all the same – well done.'

'Sure you weren't hiding in the bagel shop?' Freya said, not breaking the handshake. 'I saw someone in there with a military coat, you know. Weren't stalking me, were you?'

He grinned. 'You going to buy me one, then?'

'I think we'd best get going. Especially if you're driving.'

'Follow me.'

Out in the car park was a pure white vintage MG. She had seen it, and immediately dismissed it. When he pulled out his keys and slid them into the lock, she cocked her head. 'Seriously?'

For the first time, Harvie looked hurt. 'What do you mean?'

'It's a gorgeous car… It's very you,' she added quickly. 'Is there going to be space for my backpack?'

'Sure. At your feet.'

The seats had clearly been re-upholstered, fitting the contours of her body beautifully. He'd clearly worked hard on this car; something of a pride and joy. *Or, oh God, he's trying to impress me.*

The engine was far too noisy as they pulled out into light traffic. Heads turned as they passed. In the close heat of the late afternoon, he triggered the window and laid his elbow on the sill. *Time marks everyone*, Freya thought. *Everyone can see the generation gap but them. Is it a delusion that kicks in in the forties, or later?* Maybe even as recently as the 1990s, this set-up wouldn't have seemed naff; might even have seemed classy. She half expected him to put on racing gloves or aviator shades.

'It's not too far,' he said. 'We're away from the main resort, out into the retirement zone. Nice place he's got.'

'Wife there with him?'

'Just him. Wife died, while he was still on the force. No one else for him since then, according to my information.' He glanced across at her lap, where she was tapping a message into her phone to Glenn. 'You got something to record him with?'

'I've brought a digital voice recorder. Don't you worry.'

He nodded. 'There's every chance you'll get a door slammed in your face. Or maybe even worse.'

'You said you were friends?'

'No I didn't. I said he was a good copper. Friends is a relative term. He was never the type of guy to leak anything to the press. A few of his lieutenants, yeah. Maybe he even put a few of them up to it. But Bernie Galvin always let you know which side of the fence you were on. As I said, I respected him.'

'So why don't you want to speak to him?'

'It'll be better all round if you do it. You're more likely to get a result than me. It'll be a surprise to him. And there's every chance he'll give the time of day to a young thing like yourself, as I've said.'

'So where will you be?'

'I'll be nearby, getting some photos. You won't even know I'm there. He certainly won't.'

'It sounds a little bit dodgy to me. What if he invites me in?'

'Then you bloody go in! He's not going to bite you. He's too old. Must be pushing seventy, now.'

Freya glanced at the wattled lines of Mick Harvie's neck, then decided not to pursue an obvious line of inquiry. 'What if he chops me up?'

He laughed aloud. 'Now that'd be a turn-up for the books, and no mistake. If it happens, well, I want you to know… you'll be front-page news.'

Bernie Galvin's bungalow was at the end of a lovely row of sugarloaf houses, all competing against each other for the most colourful floral display. It hurt Freya's eyes to look at the yellows, pinks, purples, and especially the reds, so bright they seemed to shimmer.

'This is where we say toodle-oo,' Harvie said. 'I'll make myself scarce. You may be tempted to look out for me in the line of trees just across the road. You have to ignore this temptation.'

Beyond the treeline was the sea. They had climbed a long way in the car without Freya noticing, until she saw some distant oil tankers hugging the horizon.

'Remember, don't get adversarial. You're trying to get his thoughts on the case. Try to coax him in. It's not a fight.'

'I think I know how to speak to someone by now, Mick. I'm a full adult.'

'All the same, you've not been in this game as long as I have. And that's almost twice as long as you've been alive. So, take a tip.'

'I'll bear it in mind.'

Harvie ducked away across the road. Freya, with her digital recorder in her pocket, approached the front door.

The gate squeaked appallingly, despite a coat of new-looking blue paint. She half expected a dog to bound down the neat little stone path towards her, but none appeared. The door was painted the same shade as the gate. It, and the frame around it, looked fresh, as did the whitewashed walls. A thatched roof might have suited this bungalow perfectly, but instead there was a topping of red tiles and a skylight.

No car was parked in front; there was no sign of life at the front windows.

Freya knocked on the door, and waited. There being no response, she knocked harder, then stood back, surveying the windows. Nothing. No sign of anyone home. The sun cast the house in a golden tone that made Freya think of dripping honey. She could think of nothing better than to stay in a house like this.

She noticed a gate at the western edge of the house. It was ajar. Freya didn't hesitate, and made towards it. As prescribed, she resisted the temptation to glance back towards the trees, now a fair distance behind her.

The gate seemed like an open invite. So, she took it. It opened out onto a perfectly kept lawn, with turf that looked like the greens on a golf course. A water feature tinkled somewhere, nearby a squat shed, painted camouflage green.

'Hello?' she called out, uncertainly. 'Mr Galvin?'

She took a step or two inside the gate. Then she heard a clear, definite click.

'Who the fuck are you?' The accent was northern, possibly Leeds, or somewhere on the periphery. It came from somewhere over her right shoulder; she dared a look, but still couldn't see anyone.

'My name's Freya Bain. I've come to see if you'll agree to an interview.'

'An interview for what, exactly?'

'Sorry, I don't know exactly who I'm talking to.'

'The person who owns this fucking house, that's who. The house you're trespassing in.' Finally, he revealed himself. He had changed a lot from the photograph Mick Harvie had shown her earlier – his hair was white, and badly thinning, and he had put on a fair amount of weight. But he still had the shoulders, the build and the hands of a prize fighter, a boxy man with a low centre of gravity – no more than five foot seven – who would have intimidated men much taller.

He also had a shotgun, pointed straight at her.

She raised her hands, pulse quickening. 'I'm not armed,' she said, ludicrously.

'I know that, Calamity Jane. Had you been armed, I'd have sprayed you over the back wall.'

'That's a shame,' she said, her throat closing up on her. 'You've just had it repainted, I can see.'

'Which paper you from?'

'The *Salvo*.'

'The *Salvo*? You know what I used to say whenever someone from the fucking *Salvo* called me up? When I was on the force? They'd say, "I'm Johnny Fuckface from the *Salvo*," and I'd say, "The *Salvo*, eh? You're fucking fired."' When Freya didn't laugh, he lowered the shotgun. 'Don't piss your pants. I won't shoot you. Unless you give me a really good reason.'

'I'm not going to give you any, um, reason to.' She lowered her hands – slowly. Her head was swimming, a curious draining sensation at her neck. She wondered if this was what it meant to faint. She shut her eyes, took a deep breath, then opened them. The world stopped spinning.

'Why'd you come in that gate?'

'Because you left it open.' She forced herself to look into his wide, hostile grey eyes. It was easier to do now that the shotgun was pointed towards the jet-washed paving stones. 'And I'll bet you did that deliberately. See me coming, did you?'

'Maybe.' A trace of a smile. It seemed an effort for him to execute one properly. His face had a corrugated look, especially around the mouth and the forehead. These were not laugh lines. 'Maybe you're not as green as you look. So, Freya Bain, from the *Salvo*. You on work experience?'

'No. I'm not staff. I'm working on a feature… On the Woodcutter case.'

'Woodcutter case. You probably weren't fucking born when the Woodcutter was about. What's going on with that, then? Fucker's still trying to claim he didn't do it. Daft bastard. Yeah, I put him away. And that's where he's staying. You can quote me on that.'

'It's him I'm here to talk about – Gareth Solomon. I'm his daughter.'

The face fell. He seemed confused, for a moment, and looked a lot older than he was. 'You're the lass in the paper the other day.'

Freya nodded.

He scowled at her a moment, then said: 'You've had a haircut since then. Changed the colour a bit. Yeah… I see his eyes, all right. I could believe that, lass.'

'I want to talk about him… I reckon that he's not the Woodcutter.'

Galvin laughed aloud; Freya flinched. 'Not the Woodcutter? Sweetheart, I don't know how well you know your daddy, but not as well as I know him. And that fucker is in the right place, let me tell you. He's a deviant, and for my money, he slaughtered all the others. And a few more besides that we don't know about. So, don't try and tell me my business.'

Freya nodded, hoping she hadn't turned her digital recorder off when she'd leapt in fright. 'I understand what you're saying. I know that he's a compelling suspect.'

'Compelling? That's one way of putting it. He's a cert. Now I don't know what this new case they're trying to link with it is, but I can tell you…'

'New case? You mean the old bodies, the ones they've found?'

'But I can tell you,' he continued, blinking, 'that he killed those five people. He took them somewhere quiet, and he hunted them down. And when he caught them, he chopped them up. He's a smart bugger, I'll say that. But Gareth Solomon is the Woodcutter. He's not getting out of jail. If there's a copycat out there, then it's nothing to do with him, I guarantee you.'

'A copycat? Sorry, how do you mean, a copycat?'

'I've said all I want to say to you. At least now, I've had a good look at you. Now, be so kind as to give your man a shout, and then be on your way. And make it fast?'

Freya then did what she said she wouldn't do; she glanced towards the trees. 'My man?'

'No, not over there.' And here Bernard Galvin raised his shotgun – using it as a pointer. 'Over there. In my garden. Other direction. The man in the trees.'

'There isn't a man in the trees,' Freya said, desperately.

'A photographer, I'm guessing. Mind you, I saw that prick Harvie's name attached to your story, the other day. One of my old boys at the nick called me to say he'd been sniffing around. In a way I hope it is him. I really do.' Galvin stalked towards the treeline at the back of his garden, near the shed. 'Come on out, son. Best if you come out,' he called, confidently.

'I'm serious – there's no one there,' Freya said.

'Interesting. Perhaps it's a third party?' Galvin grinned. 'We're going to find out who it is, anyway.' And he bellowed: 'Whoever's in there. You've got to the count of five. Then I start shooting. One...'

The trees rustled. There was an impression of a spindly-limbed spider detaching itself from one of the branches; then a figure dropped to the ground, in front of the back fence, straightened up, and walked towards them.

30

Bernard Galvin's tongue protruded in a grotesque leer as the man in the trees came into view. 'And here he is, the man for all seasons. Come on down.' He cackled. 'The rural life suiting you all right, Harvie?'

'Put the gun down, Bernard,' Mick Harvie said, striding through the trees. His hands were raised. 'No one means you any harm, here.'

'Oh, I'm well aware of that.' Galvin rested the shotgun in the crook of his elbow. 'If I thought you meant me any harm, you'd be dead already. I was just explaining that to the young lady, here.'

'You know who she is?' Harvie's face was set, tense.

'She mentioned it.' Galvin moved a little closer to his shed – only a few paces away from Harvie, but at an improved angle to keep them both covered. He studied Freya closely, now. The sense of gruff amusement faltered a little. 'Yeah, now I see her in this light… Little doubt about it. You're his daughter all right, lass. I don't need to see any DNA test results to know it. God. How does that *feel*?'

'No one's asked me that yet,' Freya said.

'Pretty sure I did,' Harvie muttered.

'Stop gibbering, both of you,' Galvin said. He gestured

towards Freya with the shotgun; she fought the urge to run. 'Now, you say you're here to ask some questions. I might even have answered a few, had I not spotted this evil little chimp scuttling around the front of the house. He working with you, I take it?'

Freya said nothing.

'I'll assume that's a yes. OK. Yeah, interesting times with the Woodcutter case. First you pop up in the papers, asking all sorts of questions… Then you find one of the bodies… Then I hear that you find another.'

Harvie frowned. 'Second body? When was this?'

Galvin chuckled. 'Listen to him! Always the innocent, is Mick Harvie. I'll give you some free advice, Miss Woodcutter Junior or whatever they call you. Don't listen to anything this sewer rat tells you.'

'Missed you too,' Harvie said. His voice was steady but Freya could discern a slight tremor in his hands.

'Aren't you two old friends?' Freya said.

'No we are not,' Bernie Galvin said, very quietly. 'Never were, never will be. Not in a million years.'

Harvie made no response to this.

'Anyway… I'll answer a couple of questions, miss… was it Freya? Yeah. Go for it. I'm in a forgiving mood, even though you're trespassing. Did you know… if you trespass in someone's house, you're giving them a right to kill you?'

'You left your gate open. I was just coming around the back of the house, to see if you were home.'

'Sure you were. Like you'd do that in anyone else's home. Y'know, the press… it's changed since my day – since the days this ferret-faced carbuncle did his thing at press conferences… All technology, now. But you people don't really change, do you? You just find new ways to invade people's privacy.'

Freya could feel the colour rising in her face. She cleared her throat, then said: 'You mentioned something else that was going on – before you mentioned the second body. What was it? What do you mean by that?'

'Don't play the fucking innocent. You, and that little Murder Supper Club you have going. What is it – Red Ink? You're up to your necks in something. You've got information coming from somewhere, and I promise you – I still know some boys, real hard nuts, the lads who were coming up in the world round about the time I dropped out. And I can promise, whatever you know, they'll get it out of you. Whether you make it easy or hard, they'll find out. And they'll find out whether you're linked to the new carry-on.'

'What carry-on? This is the bit I don't get. What new stuff do you mean?'

'The body they found. Or, the bits of the body they found. Oh come on! All those access to sources you boast about, and you don't fucking know? You will, in about twenty-four hours.'

'Are you trying to tell me that they've found another body? Out of the final two that're missing?'

'Jesus, maybe you don't know. Well, you'll soon find out.' He smirked.

'Slow down a minute,' Harvie said to her. 'Unless my maths is out, you're telling me that you've found another one of the missing bodies? In the space of a few fucking days? And you didn't think to tell me?'

'You didn't ask,' Freya said simply.

'We'll talk about this later,' Harvie growled.

'Don't talk to the lady like that,' Galvin told him, again, in the peremptory tones of a bored, experienced teacher who yearned for the days of corporal punishment. 'Hey, Freya – whatever he's promising you for these gigs at the *Salvo*, I promise you he'll be on at least double. Tip for you – call the office, make a few inquiries, speak to accounts, if it isn't run by a spreadsheet these days. He's probably diddling you. He diddles everyone, when he can.'

'Isn't that the truth,' Harvie said, pointedly. 'You know who I've diddled, all right.'

There was a terrible silence for a moment. 'I could do it, you know,' Galvin said, quietly. 'End you with one pull of the trigger, here. I'm fully licensed, in case you're wondering. If I did both of you, know what would happen? Know what action would be taken?' He moved a step towards Harvie. To his credit, the latter held his ground. 'Fuck all,' Galvin said, at last. He aimed the shotgun at Harvie's neck. Freya hardly dared move.

'Murder, Bernard? That what you're all about, here?' Mick Harvie appeared to be losing control of his voice; it fluctuated between high and absurdly high. 'Thought you were one of the good guys.'

'I don't know about one of the good guys. I just know I'm not a prize bastard like you, son.' Nonetheless, Galvin lowered the weapon.

'Second question,' Freya asked. 'Carol Ramirez. Why is she difficult to find?'

'There's a reason for that,' Galvin said. 'She's mentally ill. She's got various diagnoses from various psychiatrists. None of them can agree with each other, but I can give you a pointer: fucking gaga, is how I'd put it. She's a 'nana. Always was.'

'Did she have an affair with my father?'

'I dunno. Ask him.'

'I think you know that she did have an affair with him. I think you know that she could have cleared him. But she was prevented from giving evidence in court. It might have cleared my dad. Everyone knows this. Can you admit it's possible that she was his alibi?'

'His slave, is what she was. Your dad, he wasn't lacking in charisma. I'll say that. You know how they reckon a sailor can have a girl in every port? He had a woman in every town he passed through. The gift of the gab. I guess you're proof of that. Somehow he managed to chat up a serving police officer, who didn't know any better because she was, as I might have mentioned, fucking crazy.'

'I see the winning manner hasn't changed,' Harvie said. He laughed at his own joke, until Galvin said: 'Don't open your mouth again until I tell you to.'

Freya said: 'When did it become obvious Carol Ramirez was "crazy", as you put it – before you knew she was involved with my dad, or after?'

Galvin stood up straight, and said soberly: 'Carol Ramirez had undergone a psychiatric assessment long before she is understood to have met your father. She made a lot of things up about him. She was quoted as saying that it was written in the stars that they should be together. She heard a prophecy through the radio and television. Read special messages in the newspapers, she claimed. Cryptic clues, voices. The spookies, aliens, whatever. By the time we arrested him, she had been signed off sick – severely ill, alarming everyone she worked with. That's the truth, and that's the official line. She would have struggled to tell the difference between day and night. That's how badly affected she was. And that's all I'm saying about Carol Ramirez. As for the alibi… it's one he put in her head. It was all awfully convenient, the way it seemed to counter every point the witness said.'

'I would say the witness was convenient. The one who saw my dad in the van.'

Galvin's face flushed. 'Your dad is a maniac. I don't know who you've been speaking to, what they've told you… He's a nutter. He tortured animals when he was a kid. Probably abused six ways from Sunday. He pissed the bed. He was a voyeur. Watched women get undressed. He had a fascination for military things, being a commando. When the army kept rejecting him, he got into a fantasy life. His fantasy was to hunt down and kill people.

'He fits the profile in every way. He had a history of violence, and manipulative behaviour. He picked up women, used them and flung them away like they were shit-rags. No offence, but it's true. He ticked every single box, and then we had a witness place him at the scene. The only bit of evidence that might have cleared him came from a headcase who told us that he was related to Jesus and was in contact with alien beings. That's not me having a laugh – that's what she told me, to my face. Quote unquote. He fucking did it, he's the Woodcutter, and that's that!'

'So you didn't fit him up?'

Galvin chewed the side of his mouth for a moment or two. 'All right, that'll do it. Get out. It should go without saying, but I don't want to see either of you around here again.'

Freya waited for Harvie to catch up with her on the garden path. Galvin followed them, the shotgun pointing towards the ground. Freya didn't want to turn her back on him; his face was flushed, and a fleck of spittle dangled from his lower lip like bad awning.

'Nice garden you've got here,' Harvie said. 'Not as good as the one in your last house, mind, but you've done a bang-up job.'

'Word of advice for you, Mick,' Galvin said. 'Just before you go.'

Harvie half-turned – and that's when the shotgun barrel smashed him across the face.

There was a dull sound of metal on flesh. Harvie barely cried out; he fell to the ground.

Galvin was on him like a cat spearing a starling. The shotgun was laid aside; his knees on Harvie's chest, he punched him once, twice, three times in the face. He drew back after the third blow, hissing breath through his teeth.

Freya ran forward, shrieking; then Galvin was off his knees and on his feet in one bizarrely fluid move, the shotgun back in his hands and pointed straight at her.

Bernard Galvin was laughing, yelping strangely in between gulping breaths. 'You know you think about doing something for years, then finally get the chance? You ever done that? I just have.'

'You're a fucking animal,' Freya said. She crouched and took Harvie by the shoulders. It wasn't clear if he was fully conscious; his eyes rolled alarmingly in his head, reminding Freya of eggs cracked into a cup. Blood dripped from his nose, mouth, and a long gash in his face, right where his beard met his cheekbone. This latter wound was already swollen.

'Bastard,' Harvie wheezed.

Then Galvin stole forward again, as Harvie sat up, planting a kick right in the apex of his splayed legs. Harvie screamed, then.

'Don't forget it!' Galvin said, savagely.

'For Christ's sake, he's had enough!' Freya said – shielding Harvie with an upraised hand. 'Leave him alone!'

'It's all right, I'm done. That's out of my system.' Galvin straightened up, his back cracking. 'Now – off you jolly well fuck.'

31

Blood dripped onto the pristine white bodywork of the MG. Mick Harvie tutted, then wiped it off with the edge of his sleeve. She noticed his hand was shaking uncontrollably.

Freya kept her distance from him. Caught between pain and humiliation, he had stalked off once they'd gotten out of Bernard Galvin's back gate, muttering to himself. She gave him a little bit of space, after making sure she had everything safely recorded on the device in her pocket. At the car, she noticed his face was still bleeding quite heavily, staining the salt and pepper beard and dipping onto the collars of his green military jacket. Freya thought of raindrops pattering the fronds of a plant in the jungle.

Galvin had come out to leer, bathing in curtain-twitching attention of his neighbours on the narrow little avenue. He had, perhaps wisely, ditched the shotgun somewhere.

'Lovely to see you again, Michael. Do come back and we'll take tea sometime.' He gave the thumbs-up sign, and grinned dementedly. From a distance his wide grey eyes seemed to glow. 'You don't even have to knock! It'll be a pleasure to see you.'

'Bastard,' Harvie snarled. 'I will make it my mission… I swear to God…'

They reached the car. Harvie's limp having grown progressively worse.

'Mick?' Freya said. 'Turn around… Please. It's all right. I just want to check you out.'

'It's fine,' he said. He actually smiled; his front teeth were smeared with blood. He ran a tongue over his teeth, frowned, then dabbed a finger against the enamel. Seeing his bloody fingertips, he spat onto the pavement. 'I've had worse. Not for a while, but… I've had worse.'

'I'm not sure I believe you. Look, you're hurt. We've got to go to the police…'

She didn't stop herself in time. Harvie laughed. 'If you want to give a statement, head on up the drive. He seems to enjoy company.'

'We should get you to casualty. It was a head injury… did you hit your head on the ground when you fell?'

'I hit my head on a few things, at high speed.' He fiddled for his keys, face pinched tight, whether in concentration or in pain, it was hard to say. At this point he looked old – properly old, the bent old man he would surely become. An inch or two shorter than he thought he was.

'Are you going to be all right to drive?'

'Don't insult me. You going back to the smoke?'

She nodded. 'Look, I think I've got a first aid kit in my bag… No offence, but I don't want you to bleed on me.'

He sighed. 'All right. I'll indulge you. Let's get in the car.'

Inside, she cleaned the cut with wipes and passed him a dab of antiseptic. He applied it the way a nun might apply blusher, then accepted a further offering of cotton wool and a sticking plaster over the top. The other side of his face was already swollen, and at closer quarters she could see his mashed lips had swollen. 'He blindsided you, Mick. Nasty move.'

'An arse-kicking is an arse-kicking. You get them in life, love. Not saying they're pleasant, but they're inevitable. Key thing is to learn from them.'

Freya screwed the cap back on the antiseptic. 'Don't go all stoic. That guy's an ex-police officer, acting like a thug. He should be in prison for that.'

'Nah, I don't grass, love. That's the law of the jungle, section one, sub-section A. Plus, we were trespassing. What he said about shooting us was true. He wouldn't even have been charged.' He stole a look in the mirror underneath his sun visor, and he winced. 'Great chance to pop him one, all the same. I'll regret that.'

'Pop him one? What are you, Bruce Lee? He had a gun, Mick.'

'Forget about it. It's done. We got what we came for. In a manner of speaking.'

'Question one, though. The way you spoke about him up till now, you'd think you were friends. You defended him when I suggested he'd gotten it wrong about my dad. You didn't look like you were friends.'

Harvie sighed. 'What I told you was true. I left out the part about me and his wife.'

'You're kidding… I mean, I picked up on that from what you said, about diddling and what have you. But I thought you were… Well, just kidding.'

'I'm afraid not. It just sort of happened. She worked with the police, too. Wasn't in uniform – liaison officer of some kind. Named adult, they called it. Nice. Everyone liked her. Marian, her name was. Marriage had been on the rocks for years. And Bernie had worked his way through a lot of women. Been a bit naughty about it – wives and girlfriends he'd met on the job. The big consoling tough guy. Could have been sacked a dozen times over, but they turned a blind eye. And that was just the ones I heard about. I'm surprised he holds a grudge, in fact.'

'You'd be surprised how far people will go to get someone back.'

'That's the truth. You know, he has no idea if it's true? I met her out on a job one day. Rough one. Child abuse case at a home. We both needed a drink, got talking…' He gestured with his hands. 'Both of us married. It got out, of course. These things do. But Bernie could never prove anything.'

'Let me guess, he deduced what you were doing? Or he followed a string of clues?'

'Or maybe his missus told him. Either way, I don't care. It happened. I don't regret it. You're young – you'll know all about it. And Marian's dead, anyway. Cancer. Quick. You'll know all about that, too.' After a moment, he added: 'Sorry.'

'S'all right. I forget, myself, every now and again.'

'Now I've got a question for you. What's this about body number two?'

Freya told him – or at least, the version of events she'd told the police only that morning. Harvie lunged forward in his seat, gripping the steering wheel. Had the car been in motion, Freya fancied that he might have swerved them off the road. 'This happened last night! And you didn't think to tell me?' He began to scan his phone. 'Nothing on the wires or any of the digital channels… Christ almighty!'

'It was a scoop, Mick.' She shrugged. 'Sometimes we have to play our cards close to our chest, in this game. You'll know all about that. You know, after you took a liberty with me before?'

He glared at her, then relaxed into a smile that almost dislodged his plaster. 'You've got the cheek, I'll say that for you. Got the patter, too. You're young and pretty enough that it won't get you into trouble. Not just yet, anyway. So that's two bodies, turned up. We're up to three. And they reckon it was Ceulemans?'

'The Dutch girl?'

'The gypsy.'

'The backpacker, I think might be the term. The girl on her gap year. Or having an adventure during the holidays.'

'Whatever. Let's deal with the facts. You can get sentimental in your one-thousand-word think piece.'

Freya bristled. 'And the facts are, if you'd let me finish, that no – they didn't find Florence Ceulemans. They think the new body was Coleen Arden's. The girl from Edinburgh.'

'So that's just two to go? And you've found 'em both?'

'Not just me. Me and Glenn.'

'Oh, the Red Ink geek. Yeah. Royal pain in the arse, that boy.'

'Good reporter. You must admit.'

'He's not in the trade. He's a pretender. Sitting at the computer with a sock on his dick. That's not a reporter.'

'He's scooped everyone on this one,' Freya mused, interested in how agitated Harvie had become at this development, considering someone had wrecked his face minutes beforehand.

'Anyway. You get more scoops… Come to me. Don't listen to him. I'll get you the money.'

'It's not about the money, Mick. I keep telling you.'

'Whatever.' He started the car, and then pulled away from the street. They both gazed in their side mirrors, perhaps both seized by the same conviction that Galvin might appear in them, aiming both barrels at the departing car. 'Anyway – no joke. Any tips you get, share them. I'll make sure you get paid.'

'What do you reckon to the other stuff he was talking about? That was kind of cryptic. Was he talking about the inquiry being opened? And did he mention a copycat?'

'That did intrigue me,' Harvie said, flicking on the indicator as they approached a roundabout.

'Is it something you know about?'

'Could be.' He smiled, as if to himself.

'Spill it, then. I'll share my scoops with you, if you tell me what you know about the inquiry.'

'I just heard one or two things. Haven't had anything confirmed, upon pain of death. And as you've had demonstrated this afternoon, that's not a one hundred per cent uncertain outcome if I cross some of my snitches.'

'Come on. What do you know?'

'There is a rumour that another body has turned up.'

'One of the other two?'

'No, not one of the Woodcutter's victims. This is another body. A new one. There are similarities in the case. But it happened quite recently. So it couldn't have been your dad. Young lass, out doing triathlon training out on a lakeside.

North of the border. Vanished. What was left of her was found near an abandoned fat-processing plant in North Yorkshire. About a week or so ago.'

'What's left of her…?'

'Chopped up. With an axe.'

'Christ. This is… I had no idea.'

'No one does, yet. Not the very gory detail. So, your hotshot friend's contacts aren't quite as good as mine. Interesting, that. Although I'll need to have a word with them about the second body being found. Never mind, though, we'll have that online within a couple of hours.'

'Yeah. Don't mention it.' Freya watched the hillsides scrolling past her for a while. 'So they reckon it's the Woodcutter, then? The same guy who did the others?'

'Doubt it. The Woodcutter's your dad. I know it. But I admit it's a remote possibility that he isn't. The other possibility is: we've got a copycat. I don't know what scares me the most.'

32

Freya swirled her chopsticks around the noodles. Perfectly sliced chicken squares, sesame oil, soy sauce, pak choi, spring onion and a good belt of ginger. It was perfect. She ate quickly, unselfconsciously.

'Sorry,' she said, to Glenn, dabbing her mouth with a napkin, 'I realised I hadn't eaten much today. Think the last half-decent dinner I had was nachos or something. At that pub.'

'You've missed a bit on your...' He gestured at the side of her mouth.

'Ah. The downside of soy sauce – but there are many upsides.'

Glenn hadn't particularly dressed up for this meeting in her favourite noodle bar. He wore a polo shirt he might have worn in the gym, ancient corduroy trousers and what appeared to be the type of old man's boat shoes you might have noted with some bemusement in the centre aisle of the cheapest supermarket out there. Seeing its chance, Freya's embarrassment slipped into the seat beside her and introduced itself. It was like a kind of sonar, a constant pinging through the whole evening.

Not a date, then, she'd thought.

'Look,' he said at last, after he'd fought with a hot 'n' sour soup for so long that the waiter indicated it was fine to leave it alone. 'I just thought we should talk about the other night. Before we go on.'

'What part of the other night? The murder bit, or...?'

'You know what bit I mean.'

'Look, if you're uncomfortable, then we can just leave it to one side. It's no problem. We were both in a stressful situation. We needed to get something out of our system. And it was fine. We can just leave it there, where it is. No need for any dramas.'

'OK. That's not quite what I was meaning, but...'

'Spit it out, Glenn.'

'I was just thinking that, after all this is done, maybe we can... We can talk about it then.' He cleared his throat. 'How about beer? I quite like these formula pilsners they do in here.'

'Beer is good.' She smiled. 'So. How was your day?'

'Bit crazy. The cops weren't happy with the blog going up, as you can imagine.'

'They come to talk to you again?'

'Yeah.'

'Tamm? Looks young, but might be wizard-frozen in time for one thousand years.'

'Yes.' He chuckled. 'That's very good. Yeah, it was him. Slippery bugger. I was trying to explain that there was no harm in me posting anything, because no one's been arrested. Technically speaking, the guy they think is the Woodcutter is still in jail, so it's not sub judice. Tamm asked me about how the victim's family might feel about that. I think he might have gotten a bit angry.'

'It's almost like he's cheesed off you scooped them, or something.'

'I've had the police all over me, anyway. Had a laptop taken away. Glad I've got a spare.'

'Jesus, it must be weird knowing they will be going through your browsing history like Nurse McLaidlaw checking for nits back in primary.'

'Like I say… I've got a spare,' Glenn said. 'And I'm very careful about sources. If they're looking for the Woodcutter, then the main point of contact is you.'

Freya caught the waiter's eye, and signalled for two beers. 'This leaves us with the cryptic clue our man left us. "Two ways". What do you reckon he meant by that?'

'It's got to be a location. Everything he's told us so far has led us to certain places. I'll get my thinking cap on.'

'I already looked up places called Two Ways… a lot of pubs, funnily enough, though I doubt he'd try that one again. Derelict or not.'

'I'll keep on it. There'll be something to go on. In the meantime… How about your disappearing act yesterday?'

Glenn had said this with some vehemence. 'Is that why you're in such a weird mood?' she asked, after a pause.

'Well, it was a bit weird to be just left holding the baby, so to speak, while you sodded off to God knows where.'

Freya's eyes sparkled as she took a drink. 'I know. I had a good reason to go, though. This is the exciting bit. You'll like this. I met Bernard Galvin.'

'You what?'

'Yep.' She related the story of the previous day's events. Glenn said nothing. He gazed at her, barely even blinking, only once moving to push his glasses back up his nose. 'It was an eye-opener. It was a face-opener, as well. You should have seen the state of Harvie after it – what an absolute mess. I shouldn't laugh, but he's all worldly-wise and I'm-a-fucking-big-tough-guy, and then…'

'I thought we'd discussed this,' Glenn said.

'What?'

Glenn folded his hands. 'We talked about this. Splitting what we know.'

She sighed. 'I'm telling you now. It only happened yesterday. Hold your horses. I thought you'd be interested in, you know, the events.'

'But you kept it a secret from me. Even after we'd gone through that.' He crunched a prawn cracker, savagely.

Freya folded, unfolded and refolded the stained white napkin on her lap. His gesture had been so petulant, she wanted to laugh. She almost expected him to hurl the soup on the floor. 'I wanted to see what Mick Harvie wanted. That's for a start. Secondly, he said it had to be me and nobody else, or the deal was off. News just in – he doesn't like you.'

Glenn's shoulders relaxed. 'Any particular reason?'

'Take your pick. You're getting scoops he couldn't get, even when he was in the game. You're part of a new media he doesn't really understand. And when men like him don't understand things, they hate it. Plus, you're clever and handsome, and for all his experience in taking down shorthand in boring court cases, you've got more scoops on the Woodcutter than he ever has. Including me. In a manner of speaking.'

He actually blushed at this praise, and refocused the subject. 'So Bernard Galvin actually pummelled him?'

'As God is my witness. I thought for a second he was going to blow Mick's head off. When he brought the gun around, I was sure he was going to open fire. He pretty much threatened us. Which was a bit daft, as I recorded every word that came out of his mouth.'

'Seriously?'

'Yep. Every word of it. He's a really nasty piece of work. Aged horribly, too. I looked at some old newspaper file pics of him back in the day – black and white, really poor grain, even for the 1990s – and he looks almost pleasant. Quite a handsome man. Still handy enough, like a boxer, you know? Middleweight, maybe. Now he looks like Goya painted him. If I hadn't stepped in, he might still be punching Mick Harvie's face into mince as we speak.'

'Jesus. That's a hell of a grudge.'

'Harvie claims he fucked his wife.' Freya shrugged. 'I suppose that tends to upset people.'

'A copper's wife! Jesus.'

'That's what I said. He was unrepentant about it.'

'You'd think he would have mentioned this.'

'Just shows you – there's always more going on than you think.' Freya swiped up the last cracker and tossed it into her mouth. 'Anyway. Adds a little bit more spice to it. My take on the whole thing, though, is that they're both converts to the theory that my dad is not the Woodcutter.'

'You know my thoughts about that.'

'And they've been duly noted. There's one other thing that's got Galvin spooked, though. Harvie told me about it. Something that was outside what they knew. Galvin let it slip while he was ranting at us. He assumed we already knew about it. But we didn't.'

Glenn sat forward in his seat. 'Go on.'

'They've found another body. Not, like, our bodies. A new one. A new case. Someone who got chopped up. An amateur triathlete or wild swimmer. She disappeared at a sea loch in Scotland. Turned up in the middle of a forest, inside, get this… a picnic hamper.'

'Chopped up?'

She nodded.

'A new case? A new Woodcutter murder?'

'Looks that way. Harvie made some inquiries, while he drove me back down south. Had it confirmed. Nothing set in stone, of course, it could be anything. But they reckon, with the other bodies being found and my dad appearing in the papers, that there is a chance…'

'Surely it's a copycat?'

'Maybe. But there's every chance it's the original. Back out of retirement. You said it yourself. BTK, was that the guy? He came out of retirement to kill again. There are one or two others who had a sabbatical, then got right back into it in middle age. Maybe seeing himself in the papers turned him on? Or maybe, like you said, he got jealous of my dad getting the attention?'

'I've heard nothing about this, nothing…' He dived for his phone. 'I'll need to get onto it. I haven't heard shit from my contacts…'

'There's something else I have to tell you,' she said.

He put his phone down. He looked genuinely frightened; she wanted to reach out and touch him. She did, folding her hand over his.

'It's nothing heavy, Glenn. Jesus, you're like a seventeen-year-old. It's about Carol Ramirez. I've got one or two contacts who work in mental health. I used to do some shifts in a care home. They've managed to track her down. I think I can get an interview with her. You want in?'

'Are you sure? A couple of people said she'd died.'

'No, she's alive. Not very well, but alive. I think I can get us in. Up for it?'

He squeezed her hand. 'You're on.'

Another voice said: 'Doesn't this look like a cosy outing?'

A woman in running gear appeared at the table. She was sweating, with her hair tied back, and patches staining her zip-top. Even without make-up, she was pretty, Freya saw, with fine fair eyebrows and huge blue eyes. They were brimming with tears.

Silence fell across the restaurant. Like a black hole drawing in light, this girl's appearance drew in every piece of attention.

Glenn didn't exactly instil any confidence in this new arrival. He leapt to his feet. 'Jools, this is my work colleague.'

'Have you started work down a fucking *brothel*?' the newcomer raved. Then she picked up Glenn's soup bowl.

'No, listen,' Freya began. Then Freya was decorated; she would estimate later, by looking at her sheer blouse, that she wore maybe thirty per cent to Glenn's twenty per cent, with the remainder dousing the gawping couple in their sixties over his shoulder.

'You know,' Freya said, to the couple, bedecked with seafood, as Glenn and the young woman fled like a pair of foxes startled at some wheelie bins, 'this isn't even the worst thing that's happened to him this week.' Then she covered her face in her hands, in pure shame, and cried.

33

'New bodies, you say? Good God.'

Solomon was slouched in his chair, set back from the table in front of the mirror, hands linked behind his head.

'You surely know about this by now,' Freya said. She held her hands perfectly flat on her own table, the better to stop them shaking. 'Cheryl Levison must have told you.'

'There's been no official announcement, has there?' Solomon said, eyes twinkling. 'I don't think there has.'

'Please don't get cute,' Freya said.

'Are we having a family row? God, this is exciting.'

'Between this and the bodies being found, surely your appeal's just a formality.'

'Not long till we find out. I tell you what, I'm going to miss these guys, here.' Solomon indicated the guards. 'These two guys in particular. I mean, look at them. Look at the physique. Look at the intensity. Look at the *devotion*.'

The guard stood beside Solomon, whose physique looked pub-honed over a great number of years, remained silent, barely even moving his eyes.

'There's a question I want to ask,' Freya said, calmly. 'Are you messing with me?'

'Messing with you?' He sat forward. 'I don't follow.'

'I get in contact with you… All these bodies start showing up. Everybody, including me, thinks this is an amazing coincidence.'

'Couldn't have been me. You're barking up the wrong tree on that one, Freya. The real Woodcutter is the man you want to look out for, there. And I mean that in a very real sense. He'll surely come after you, if he's active again. You have to be careful from now on. If you appearing in the papers is the spark, then the end point is you, surely. You'll be the prize.'

'It couldn't have been you, no… But it could be something to do with you.'

'If you've got any names, let's hear them. I'm as in the dark as you,' he said.

'Is it someone you know, do you think? Someone who might want to reclaim his crown after you stole it from him?'

'That's a very interesting theory. And I met a few psychos along the way – when I was in care, when I was on the roads… Some very dark, dark people out there, Freya. But none I ever suspected was an actual maniac. So no, no obvious candidates, as far as I know. All I know is, this person who's been dropping bodies here and there is doing me a big, big favour. He's showing the world what we already know. That I didn't do it. They got the wrong man. They've punished me for nothing. *Nothing*.' Solomon's voice swelled, causing some distortion in the speaker system. The two guards on either side of the mirror shared a glance, but neither made a move.

'Maybe when you come out, they'll come after you,' Freya said.

He grinned. 'Then we've got each other's backs, haven't we?'

Freya wanted to recoil from this. It must have showed, because his eyes dropped. She imagined him turning up at her door, grinning, a plastic bag full of belongings and clothes twenty-five years too small for him. 'I guess we'll have to keep our eyes peeled.'

'You look kind of tired,' he said, suddenly. 'When you taking a day off? Been working hard, I take it?'

'After a fashion.'

'What is it you do again? I forget.'

'It's not that you forgot – I didn't tell you. You could say I'm freelancing. I want to get to the bottom of this. I want to know the truth.'

Solomon folded his arms. 'Last time I'm pretty sure you said you believed me. That you knew I didn't do it.'

'I don't think you're the Woodcutter. But you might know who is. It's all very… personal. Isn't it?'

'Could be. Could just be an obsessive. The real Woodcutter could be retired with his feet up; these new killings you've mentioned, those could be down to a copycat. You ever thought about that?'

'It's one theory. I've got an open mind.'

'You should join the police. They need open minds, in there. Once you're done freelancing. What was it you did before freelancing?'

'Didn't I already tell you?'

He shook his head, and left a silence for her to fill.

'Well, I worked in the pub alongside Mum for years.'

'At the pub?'

'Yeah.'

'Gads, you must have needed prick repellent, love, if it's the same pub I remember. Either that, or you were very spoiled. Depends on your viewpoint.'

Freya ground her back teeth. 'If you get out, try not to speak to women like that.'

'Like what?'

'Like you're in a tabloid newspaper. Things have changed since the 1990s.'

'One question... is *Loaded* still a thing?'

'*Loaded*? What's that?'

'Now you're frightening me.' He sighed, and drummed his fingers on the table. 'I apologise. You're right. In my head it's still 1994. Which is year zero for you. Literally. I think Oasis are kind of a new thing. I have to remind myself Alan Shearer's not playing football any more.'

'Was he the prime minister?' She smiled. 'Joke.'

'Very good. So, you've only ever worked in the pub, alongside dear old Mary? You didn't do any qualifications, university, that kind of thing?'

'No. I didn't do well enough at school. And I didn't want to move, either.'

'That's odd. Why not?'

'I didn't want to leave Mary alone.' It was true, and admitting it brought something welling up into her throat. She took a second or two. 'And maybe I didn't want to be away from her, either. I was happy at home, I suppose. We were a team. We were as close as you can get. I never wanted a career. At first, anyway.'

Solomon ran a hand over his scalp, and closed his eyes. 'If I've been insensitive, Freya... I am truly sorry. I forget you're grieving. I know what grieving's like, you know. Not for the dead – for the missing. For my brothers and sisters. For my ma, heading out the door. The faces I knew from my earliest days, taken away from me. I know about grief. Not quite the same as yours, but it's there. So – you're a homebody. That makes two of us, I guess.' He gestured to the walls on either side.

That brought a smile from his daughter. 'Yep. I'm very set in my ways, I suppose.'

'How about friends?'

'I find this hard to admit but… I didn't make too many of those. I don't feel shy, but I'm quiet. I don't trust people that much. I had a few friends at school, but I stopped getting invited to parties. There was some gossip about me being a tramp, a street kid. There's a stigma in not having a father around. None of the other girls in my school were in that position. It was hard… I went into myself. Friday nights would be spent working at the pub. Sunday nights, we'd have a takeaway and gossip and bicker in front of the telly. Me and my mum. It's not really clear in my mind that it's gone. That I won't be able to do that any more.'

'Boyfriends, though?' he asked, brightly. 'Must have been a few of those. Or girlfriends. Yes, I know that things have changed outside, and that's all cool, now. I'm not that badly informed. Bottom line, you're a pretty girl. These two gorillas – their jaws dropped the first time they saw you, and that's a fact!'

The big guy nearest her father blushed to the roots of his shirt collar. Freya dared not look in the face of the guard stood next to her.

'I had some boyfriends, if you have to know… But no one serious. One boy went away to university. He wrote, but it fizzled out. I knew some guys at the pub, but no one nice. No lack of interest, but… it's a pub, you know? You get used to the last orders chancers and the sleazebags. You get to recognising them from the way they walk towards the bar… the way they make eye contact. It's tiresome. It was the main reason I left the pub. Left Mary to it… She loved it, you know. Working at that pub. It was life for her, as well as a job. But I had to go, I knew that much. I got a couple of college qualifications at night, then I got a job as a carer's assistant at a home.'

'That's interesting – old folks, or mad folks?'

'Old folks. It was a great job, I loved it, but… Parts of it were getting overwhelming.'

'I suppose there's only so many bums you can wipe before you get bored. Or corpses to lay out.'

Freya's heartbeat engulfed the silence for a moment or two, before she cleared her throat and said: 'I was only there a year, but it was enough. It was an eye-opener. After that, Mum got ill. I covered for her at the pub then… Well. She faded fast, after the first round of chemo didn't take care of it. You said yourself, you've seen how it goes. There's a point where they go over a cliff.'

'I don't mean to upset you.'

'No, it's fine. I don't mind telling you this. Cheaper than therapy, right?' Freya brushed a tear away from her cheek. What came next surprised even her: 'I cling to people, I know that. If I'm telling the truth, I did that with some boys. I wrote to that poor guy at university. I didn't take the hint when he didn't answer the texts. I didn't take the hint when he didn't write back. I didn't take the hint when he didn't visit me when he came back from the holidays. Someone told me he's engaged, now. So I guess I'm sad. I'm lonely. I could have just stayed at home, sat by my mum's side till kingdom come. Cancer had other ideas. So here I am. Truth be told, I'm worried I'm going to throw myself at another boy, who's bloody useless. So that's it. That's me. That's your daughter.'

'That's time up,' said the guard, quietly.

Solomon raised a finger. 'Oh, you've got to come back. Come back soon. The appeal's going to be heard… I didn't tell you about me. That's next. All about me. Come back, all right? Please?' There was a pathetic tone to his voice she hadn't heard before; without thinking about it, she nodded, and stood up.

'Sure. See you next time. Dad.'

34

They both spoke at the same time: 'Look, I…'

'Listen, Freya…'

She paused to let Glenn speak. They were in a quiet compartment of an early train. It was a horrible day outside, the worst of all conditions – summer heavy and muggy, and raining all day. Their shoes had squeaked on the platform before they'd got on the train.

'Look, I just… I didn't mean for things to get weird.'

'I wouldn't call things weird, Glenn. Disastrous, maybe. Shameful, well… Embarrassing, definitely.'

'I'm… sorry.'

When he spoke, she noticed a cut at the corner of his mouth. You had to look closely to be able to see it; it wasn't obvious but it was right at the corner, in an awkward spot. His tongue kept creeping towards it.

'Did she hit you?' Freya asked.

'No,' he said quickly. But he didn't look in her eyes. 'Just kind of shoved me, a bit. I was shouting; things got a bit heated.'

'She shouldn't be lifting her hands to you. I'm a bit less sorry now.' She sighed. 'I can't blame her either. God's sake, Glenn! I didn't know about her. You never said. Never even hinted at it. I am *disgusted* with you. I never meant to cause any harm. I never meant to have any upset. I thought you were single.'

There was an awkward silence. 'I think she's gone. It'd been finished for a while – I know that's not an excuse. It's like she knew, you know? I didn't say anything. I thought I was calm when I got home. But she knew what I'd done. In that way they know. I couldn't rule out she was following me. She's that type. She put two and two together, and…'

'Got four. How long were you together?'

'Two and a half years.'

'First girlfriend.'

'Well, no, I had girlfriends before, just not a live-in girlfriend.'

'Yeah. That's what I said. First girlfriend.'

'OK.' He relaxed a little. 'I suppose that's fair.'

'I'm not going to beat you up about it. But you did a terrible thing. I am not a cheat, Glenn.'

'So… how do we move on? We've got work to do. We've got a deal. Don't we?'

Freya didn't answer. She drummed her hands on the tabletop. 'I've got an idea. We'll do a cup of tea and a flapjack, when the guy comes along with the trolley. You look like you've been ill or something. Once we take in those oaty-sugary calories, I promise you we'll feel a whole lot better. Then we're going to talk tactics and carry on with what we were doing.'

Glenn closed his eyes. Perhaps he was wishing this situation away, she thought. Then he opened his eyes. 'I've been thinking about Harvie and Galvin…'

'Harvie was naïve,' Freya said. 'He thought he could get

the drop on a guy who'd been with the police his whole life. The guy probably invented surveillance techniques we can't even imagine.'

'The papers are onto me, now. I got door-stepped. Just as I was carrying out my stuff from the flat. Perfect tabloid situation, I suppose. They were asking about the Woodcutter.'

Freya frowned. 'Wait, she threw you out?'

'It seemed the right thing to do.'

'Where you staying?'

'A friend's.'

Freya took a deep breath. 'God. What a mess. Never mind. Which paper was it?'

'Not sure… maybe the *Salvo*. I said I had no comment. Pushed through. It was weird to be in one of those situations you see on the telly. You never think it'll be you. I just pushed past the guy. I think there was a photographer.'

'Suppose we have to get used to it. We're news, now. You looked at the hit count on Red Ink lately?'

'Yeah.' He smiled for the first time that day. 'I have to say business is good. What's next, though?'

'I guess you won't have had time to think much about "Two Ways"?'

'A few candidates. Struggling to whittle it down. Mainly pubs, like I said. Live ones, that is.'

'Tamm might be having the same ideas,' Freya mused.

'He been in touch with you?'

'No.'

'Me neither.'

Freya brightened up. 'Listen… You hear that rattle? Here's the guy with the teas and coffees.'

'Yeah, I think I'm in the mood now. You reckon the police will be following us?'

'Tamm was keen to tell me that they don't have the time or resources to follow us. Which makes me almost certain that he was lying, and we're being tailed. Anyway. It's not the police I'm worried about, now.'

'The new case?'

'Yeah.'

'Whoever this guy is, Woodcutter or no, someone wants us to find the bodies. I don't think that person wants to kill us.'

'He's going to a hell of a lot of trouble. Anyway. Let's focus on the now.' Freya turned to the man pushing the trolley through the empty carriage, and beamed at him. 'A nice cup of tea, a great big mocha, and two of your most absolutely sinful flapjacks, please, when you're ready.'

It looked like the type of country house that should have a body in the library. Neo-gothic, red brick, worth tens of millions, but left to the NHS by a millionaire with either no heirs or extremely disappointed ones. It was only when they got closer that they saw the secured windows, and the reception desk through the glass doors at the front.

'Some pile,' Glenn said. 'I'm just a little bit nervous about this, I have to tell you.'

'It does look like a haunted house,' Freya said, 'I'll give you that.'

'No, not that. I mean – is this fraud?'

'Don't worry about it.' Freya spoke out of the side of her mouth.

'I can't help it. If we get caught with this, we could be going to jail. Pretending to be a relative? It's a crime.'

'Stop talking, Glenn. We're going to talk to the woman, not rob her. It's something I have to know. *We* have to know, for sure.'

'Why won't you tell me who got you the ID?'

'It's tricky. After the care home, I worked in data capture, too. There's an awful lot of things you can do with certain connections. Tell you what – if I don't tell you any details, then there's nothing for you to tell the police about. So far as you know, this is legit. You don't have to pretend to be anybody. Except my boyfriend.'

'That's been problematic, up til now.'

'Just smile, then. And hold my hand.' Freya took his hand. Inside, though, she was squirming. Heading into lies, deceit… It sickened her, much as the situation frightened her. She saw herself simply dissolving upon questioning, racked with sobs. She even wondered, at the last moment, whether or not it was too late to turn back. There was just one thing driving her on; one single goal.

To know whether Gareth Solomon was the Woodcutter or not.

The receptionist greeted them warily.

'Hi there,' Freya said. 'I'm Stacey Broward. I'm here to see Carol Ramirez. We have a visit booked.'

The common room looked out onto the back lawn. Glenn stared out at people playing tennis on a back court. Others – of all ages and all genders – were playing pétanque.

'Not what I expected,' Glenn said, resting his hand on his chin. 'I was thinking... people in gowns. Attendants.'

'Women chained up in the attic?'

'I'm guessing I'm prejudiced. It's a nice place.'

One of the nursing staff came in, a severe-looking woman with short, stiff, white hair. 'Hi... Is it Stacey?'

Freya got up to shake hands. For a second it looked as if the nurse wouldn't respond; she took Freya's hand reluctantly.

She turned to Glenn. 'And you are...?'

'I'm Glenn. Her fiancé.'

The nurse ignored him, turning back to Freya. 'I don't know your face. How long is it since you last saw your...?'

'Seven and a half years.'

'Her condition has deteriorated since then.'

'She's not dangerous, is she?' Freya tried to sound appropriately querulous; not a difficult stretch. 'I mean, if she is...'

'If she was dangerous you wouldn't be seeing her. No, she has a complex condition, and it's well-managed. She's not even dangerous to herself. But she can be erratic.'

'I'm sure we'll be fine,' Freya said. 'I'm looking forward to seeing her.'

'It'll be good for her – Carol doesn't get many visitors. But let's not be doing anything that upsets her.'

Glenn cleared his throat. 'We'll try not to. Maybe in return, you could treat us like we're not six years old?'

'Excuse me?' Now the nurse noticed him.

'What's wrong with her, exactly?' Glenn asked. 'If it's complex, explain it to us.'

'I'm not at liberty to tell you that.'

'Paranoid schizophrenia? Psychosis? What? Is it something we should know about?'

'I am not at liberty to disclose a patient's medical details to you.'

'It's fine,' Freya said, raising a hand to stop him. 'We're absolutely fine. It's all good.'

'As I said,' the nurse continued, 'try not to do or say anything that upsets her. We'll be monitoring her, but there's nothing for you to worry about.'

'Thanks,' Freya said.

'Take a seat, we'll be with you shortly.' The nurse took an extra few seconds to glower at Glenn, before heading back out the door.

'I'm not reassured,' Glenn said. 'Are you reassured?'

Freya lowered herself into her seat, and tried to compose herself. She said, under her breath: 'That wasn't smart. When we're trying to ingratiate ourselves with people, you don't piss them off, Glenn. Smile. Act natural. Or your nearest equivalent, if you don't quite get "natural".'

'Hey, I didn't like the tone. It felt like she was giving us a security briefing. I don't want Norman Bates' ma charging in here with a lawnmower, or something.'

Freya glanced at him sharply. 'Murder website? Crime scenes? Criminal profiles? Christ's sake, Glenn. You should know that you don't get people with a split personality like that. Things aren't that simple.'

'A joke.' He raised a hand, genuinely chastened. 'To lighten the atmosphere. To make you smile.'

'Plus – if we're here visiting a relative, then it might be safe to assume that we already know what her condition is. You've just given her a hint that we don't know – so we might not be relatives. Let's hope that Nurse Ratched is an authoritarian on the not-very-clever end of the spectrum.'

'A relative, you say.' He blinked. 'You're pretending she is your *relative*?'

'Maybe it's best if you let me handle the talking.' She folded her arms, furious.

The door opened, and the nurse returned. The latter's demeanour had completely changed; her mouth had been a compressed line of disdain before, and her eyes polished glass; but now Freya and Glenn could see her teeth, either very new or dentures, in a broad, friendly smile, her eyes crinkled in mirth at a comment they hadn't heard. 'In you come, Carol.'

The woman who came in was extremely tall and slim – Freya would have said she had the body of a teenager, lithe and long-limbed. Black leggings accentuated her thin bones, while the white T-shirt over the top reminded Freya of disinterested PE kits from her own schooldays. However, the face at the top of a long, elegant neck was not that of a teenager.

Freya knew that Carol Ramirez was fifty-four, and while this age seemed horrifically advanced, Freya was old enough to appreciate that it wasn't old… or *old* old, anyway. Even so, Carol Ramirez's face was a shock; she could have been at least twenty years older. The texture of her skin was odd, as if someone had smoothed out the foil wrapper of a sweetie, and she was gaunt, with it. Her grey hair was still long, but scraped back into a ponytail, and it was hard to guess when it had last been washed. She still had the cheekbones, but everything else was sunken and hollowed. Freya was reminded of an old soul she'd passed on the street a few times as she'd biked into work. The old dear had been singing utterly ancient music hall songs, shuffling her feet at a patch between two trees on a broad shopping thoroughfare. She was selling plastic roses. The old lady hadn't stayed there long.

Carol Ramirez's eyes were pin-sharp, though. Not big, but dark, black blotted ink on white sheeting. In just one look, Freya could discern the striking young woman in uniform, familiar from the mugshot on Red Ink.

This was the most dangerous moment. Carol Ramirez stopped, and her eyes narrowed.

Then she said: 'Oh. Stacey. God, you've *changed*.'

35

'I know,' Freya said, pointing to her blonde hair, 'I can't settle. I went coal black for a while.'

'Coal black suits you. You'll get roots, going that blonde. Takes effort.'

Freya came forward. Carol looked discomfited, but Freya was undaunted. She wrapped the taller, older woman in a hug. There was little warmth in it, but Carol's hands came around to Freya's shoulders.

'You're skinnier than I remember, too,' Carol said. Her eyes were watering, twin points of light in the dark. 'Eating all right, I hope?'

'Eating plenty. I've been training a lot. Running, mostly. Been doing a fair bit of country walking, haven't we?' Freya turned to Glenn, and he nodded, earnestly.

'I don't know you,' Carol remarked.

'I'm Glenn.' He came forward, proffering a hand.

Carol Ramirez took it, as awkwardly as it was possible to shake someone's hand. Its equivalent would have been trying to high-five someone and missing, or handling something unpleasant snarled in a drain, even with rubber gloves on.

'Glenn what?'

'Glenn's my fiancé.' Freya took to his side, slithering an arm around his shoulder and drawing him close. Glenn's hand rested in the curve of her hip. This tingled, treacherously. 'That's why we came to see you.'

Carol's eyes narrowed. 'Can I see the ring?'

'Well, we...' Glenn began, but Freya came forward, tilting her left hand.

Carol took it, and scrutinised the simple ring Freya wore. There was no stone; only a hint of silver.

'Hmm. I'm guessing Glenn isn't a big spender?' At the thunderstruck silence that followed, Carol cackled, a grin splitting her face.

'Well, umm, that's just a placeholder,' Glenn said. 'The actual ring will have a rock so big you could escape from here with it.'

Carol laughed harder, delighted. 'He's cheeky – he'll do for me! Where'd you find him, love? Did you order him online?'

The nurse drew back, seemingly relieved. 'I'll leave you guys to it. You need anything, just holler.'

'There'll be no need to holler,' Carol said. 'Nurse Patterson here will be watching on the video cameras, along with a couple of strapping young men who took me over to this wing. When I spring into the attack, they'll be in here before I can do too much damage.' She smiled sweetly at the nurse.

'Take care, Carol,' Nurse Patterson said, dryly, then withdrew.

'Sit yourselves down,' Carol said. She nodded towards one of the empty tables and chairs. 'I'd say, "Help yourselves to water and the tea machine," but the last time I tried the tea it took the enamel off my teeth.'

They declined the offer, and sat down with Carol at the table.

'So – how's it been?' Freya asked.

'Oh, so-so.' Carol shrugged her shoulders theatrically. 'You know the drill. Take the pills. Wander through the day in cotton wool. A couple of times I made friends. I had a boyfriend, you know.'

'Yeah?'

'Yeah. He died.' Carol sighed, and leaned back in her chair. 'It happens. He was old, and mad. He had money and property, you know. I could have robbed him blind, but, well, he was a lunatic, and there was no chance of me getting him to change his will.'

Freya took this in her stride. 'That's the way it goes.'

Carol turned to Glenn. 'Do you have money and property?'

'I've got a decent collection of *2000AD* comics. Only one or two gaps.'

'Big fire risk, those. You'll come out like an overdone chicken when they find you, boy. Even down to the joints. I've seen it, you know. Seen it all. When I was in the police. Whatever they find clutched in your blackened hands, it won't be fucking comics. That's what they got me for, you know. I set fire to some old flats. I saw the boarded-up windows, thought they were empty. Turned out there were people still in there. Whoops!'

Glenn cleared his throat. Freya shot him a look, and he stayed silent.

'Nobody died, mind. I didn't get charged. They fix that for you, the cops. Still got sectioned, but never went before the courts. Doesn't look good to have a serving member of the constabulary go off her head. Never knew that, did you?'

'I didn't,' Freya said.

'You don't look shocked, mind. What do you know about me?'

'I'm not here to talk about that stuff,' Freya said. 'I don't think it's going to make anyone feel better.'

'Bollocks,' Carol said, brightly. 'There's something you want. I don't know you too well, but I do know you. Hey, Glenn – is she this bad a liar when she tells you she loves you?'

'She's a brilliant liar,' he said. 'She convinces me every time.'

Carol cackled again. 'I do like him. He'll do. He might be just what you need, girl. So… tell me a story, kid. What's been happening with you?'

'So far, so boring,' Freya said. 'I'm still at the call centre. It's steady enough.'

'Thought you might be one of the clever ones,' Carol said. 'You were quiet, I remember that much about you. Whenever they brought you along. I thought you were one of these deep characters. Read a lot, you know. Might go on to do something with your life, if only you'd raise your voice. I think it turned out that you were just very dull. You seem to have a bit more of a spark about you now, though. Not shy, are you?'

'We all change.'

'That's the truth. So. You going to say what you want then?'

'Is the idea of me getting engaged not enough?'

'Yes, yes. On top of that. What do you want?'

Glenn leaned forward. Before Freya could stop him, he said: 'Look, Ms Ramirez, I don't want to take up your time. We're here to learn more about a man you knew. Years ago. His name was Gareth Solomon.'

If the name had any effect on Carol Ramirez, she covered it up with something that might have been a cough, or a "hem". She leaned back and folded her arms, shifting her gaze between Freya and Glenn. 'Gareth Solomon, you say. That's not what people call him.'

'The Woodcutter, then, if you like.'

'Know him personally, do you, son?'

'I've never had the pleasure.'

'I did.' She grinned. 'It's been a while since people asked me about him. The powers that be aren't too keen on me talking about that guy.'

'Which powers that be?' Glenn asked.

Carol gestured vaguely around the walls. 'Oh, all of them. But mostly the force I used to work for. Have you ever heard of a man called Bernard Galvin?'

'That rings a bell,' Freya said.

'I bet it does. He's a bit before your time. But he was the Dirty Harry of his day. Hmm. Blank looks… I forget, time's getting on. You might not know who Dirty Harry is. Hey, is Clint Eastwood still alive?'

'Was he your boss?' Freya asked. 'Bernard Galvin, not Clint Eastwood.'

'He was everyone's boss. He ran the Woodcutter inquiry. You might want to look it up. My name's all over it, so they tell me. On the internet. They never let me go on the internet. Imagine that – you just call up a name or a face and it tells you everything you could ever want to know about them. When I was your age we had a thing called Teletext, and that seemed like space age stuff when it came out.'

'You were saying about Bernard Galvin?' Glenn asked.

'I was taking my time, son.' She didn't look at Glenn with quite so much amusement, now. The look was back; the still, fixed glare. Twin stars in negative. Freya wondered what it must have been like to have been arrested by this woman. 'Bernard Galvin was the hero cop who pulled Gareth in. Made the arrest personally. June Caton-Bell, that's another name to look up. That's the name of the last one. The one they arrested Gareth Solomon over. Anyway, old Bernard quite likes me being in here. Don't get me wrong – I deserve to be in here. But it's all good for Bernard. All good for his inquiry. He's the powers that be. Still is, for all I know. If he's still alive.'

'Why's it good news for him?'

'Because I can prove him wrong, that's why. I can prove that Gareth Solomon didn't kill June Caton-Bell.'

'Seriously?' Glenn said.

'Serious as you like. A lot of people said Gareth and me were boyfriend and girlfriend… You know, like you two are. But it's not as simple as that. We couldn't last, we both knew that. We were both into slightly different things. He liked the old tiesy-upsy. I liked… well, different things.'

There was a pause. Freya filled it. 'Different things like… what?'

'Sure you want to know? You both look so young. Oh well, better out than in. Have you ever seen the scene of a crime?'

Neither of her visitors answered.

'Sometimes you used to see photos. I saw lots. I had access to the Black Room, where they kept all the meaty ones. I don't know what it is about it exactly, but maybe I could put it like... You know when you go to a crime scene, the atmosphere is like... church. That solemn way, you know? Like you can't laugh. Did you ever laugh in church? Did either of you go to church?'

'Once or twice,' Glenn said.

'Then you must have laughed. When you were in with your friends, at school. Lamb of God, this. Body and blood, that. I know about body and blood, all right. First time I saw a dead person, their skin had turned black like liquorice, and they had swollen to about twice the size you would expect. They looked ripe. Smelled it, too. You ever see a body like that?'

Freya shook her head.

'With murders it's worse. It's like when you see trees uprooted, after a storm. The storm's gone by the time we show up, usually, but when you see the trees all slanted, and parts of a house here and there, and cars on their sides... it suggests the power to you. It suggests the storm. I can't explain it any better than that. So, when one day I came into a house where an old lady had been strangled, by her own son, it turned out... Well. I can't tell you.' She wiggled her eyebrows. She licked her lips.

'Turned you on,' Freya said, before she could fully process it. 'Is that what you mean? It turned you on.'

'Got it in one. We've all got a thing, I suppose. Something that tickles you, right where you live. That's mine. I can say this to you. I'm not bothered that you know. It's the drugs, I suppose.'

Freya felt a storm of revulsion convulsing her breast, and also… disappointment? Something more subtle? She saw the fantasy father again, the man she'd go to the seaside with. The man who would skim stones with her, and buy her an ice cream. A man who had gone dark again; a grinning shadow, with piercing eyes. She shook her head. She didn't want to believe it. 'That's not right.'

'Oh, it's absolutely awful and disgusting,' Carol said, nodding fervently. 'No question, there.'

The door opened, and Nurse Patterson came in. 'Everything OK, Carol?'

'Everything's fine,' Carol said brightly. 'Me and my family are just catching up.'

'Just five minutes more. You've got an art class today, remember.'

'Of course.' Carol smiled pleasantly. 'I'm enjoying the chat, though. It's been good.'

'I'll be back in five minutes,' Nurse Patterson said, before going out again.

Carol said out of the corner of her mouth, 'We'll need to whisper.'

'When did you meet Gareth Solomon?' Freya asked.

'There was a ruck at the pub he had been working in. He helped me deal with a tricky customer – a young guy who'd been throwing bottles around. I didn't need the help, truth be told. Gareth was more keen than anything else. It's the closest you get to normal attraction in people like us. We got talking, we got together… It was a fleeting thing, he was clear about that. But he gave me something no other man could. He said, he could show me a body. And he did.'

'When was this?' Glenn asked. His throat clicked as he spoke.

'I told you. Round about the time of the last Woodcutter case. The one they caught him for: June Caton-Bell. Lovely-looking girl, to go by the pictures. Less so when I saw her.'

'I don't understand,' Freya said, trying to keep her voice low. 'You saw the body? He took you to see the body?'

'Yep. Right there under the stars. You ever seen fresh blood by torchlight? Already had the flies setting on it, but so bright. Stained all the greenery. Hell of a contrast, under torchlight. Red and green. Black and silver. Doesn't look unnatural, though. Yeah, he knew where the body was. He took me out there. And that's when we did it, for the last time. You two are engaged, so you'll know... When you hit that peak with another person. You can't fake it. If you take away the body at the scene, we could have been normal lovers... Normal people. Doing something absolutely wonderful. Two bodies welded together. Maybe entwined is a better word, branches twisted together in a knot. We might never have separated. But Jesus Christ, the mess that was made of that girl. Whoever did that... You had to look closely to tell it was a person at all. Chopped to *pieces*. Then chopped into more pieces. Family-sized tin of tomatoes, with a couple of eyeballs in there. Splat! The strength it must have took... the sheer rage. For all we knew, he was still there, somewhere. Maybe he was watching us – who knows?'

'Wait a minute,' Glenn said. His mouth was twitching; he was close to something, a breakthrough. He could barely contain a sense of excitement; she laid a hand on his twitchy arm, to soften his voice. *Maybe this is* his *thing*, she thought. 'You're saying that Gareth Solomon knew where June Caton-Bell's body was, in the woods? He took you out there. You were together at the scene, on the spot. But you say he *didn't* kill her? You know this?'

'Know it for a fact. Gareth Solomon didn't kill that girl.' Carol smiled.

'How?'

'Because he was with me the entire day. We didn't leave the house. We had a nice late lunch, had a couple of drinks, and that's when he told me. He knew where June Caton-Bell's body was. He didn't go anywhere that day; I can tell you that for a fact. Dawn till dusk. The only time he went to the woods, he was with me. And there's no chance he stole away anywhere. He didn't sneak out for a quick five minutes, kidnap her sixty miles away, then come back.'

'But she was killed that night,' Glenn said. 'The night the woman saw him going into his van. She was killed *that night*. The body was found a couple of hours after she was killed. How could he know where the body was if he didn't kill her?'

'I can't tell you that. He's the only one who can answer that. But I can tell you that he didn't kill her. No word of a lie.'

Freya said: 'You could clear him. You could have cleared him in court.'

'True, but they'd already banged me up in here, by that point. Fully certified, doolally. And they were bang to rights. I mean, I was *fucking*, right at the scene of a murder. With the prime suspect, it turned out. Stepping back out of myself, I would have to say that's pretty messed up. On a par with actually having chopped a girl up. Wouldn't you agree?'

'You were sectioned – when?'

'I burned the house a few days after Gareth was arrested. And to be fair, they were already investigating me. It seems our internal investigations bureau had a decent file on me. It all started when some nosy bugger got curious about the amount of time I was looking at old crime scene photos. And you'd have to be a weirdo to look at those, wouldn't you, son?'

Glenn didn't seem to be aware of any irony in Carol's remark. 'Is it possible you were sectioned to take you out of the inquiry? To make sure you didn't testify in court?'

'Got it in one. Bernard Galvin needed a result. Five murders on his patch, he was under pressure. Bit of ego in there, too. You don't run a team of detectives without it. Imagine being the guy remembered as the copper who didn't catch the Woodcutter. Imagine that? He fitted Gareth up for June Caton-Bell. No question. But it does beg a question why Gareth knew where the body was going to be, possibly even before the body got there. Doesn't it?'

'What do you reckon?' Freya said, checking her watch. 'He wasn't the Woodcutter? Who was?'

'No idea, Stacey. None at all. But I wouldn't rule out Gareth as having been the Woodcutter. That'd be silly. I think he knows who killed June Caton-Bell. I think he knew they were planning to do it, whoever they were. So he didn't kill her – he couldn't have. But he probably knows who did.'

'He must know who the real killer is,' Glenn said.

'Sure he does. And he might have done some of the murders. After all, he told me where the other bodies were.'

'You what?' Freya said.

'Oh yeah. Look for where the water goes two ways.

I'll say this about Gareth Solomon – he might have been the Woodcutter. He might not. Someone else might have done all the killings. They might not.' She yawned. 'Now, I'm getting bored. Was that what you wanted, Stacey? That good enough? Now, if you'll excuse me, I'll have a hit of the good stuff.'

She lunged. Freya and Glenn sprung to their feet, both chairs falling back against the floor. But Carol Ramirez did not spring at them. She bit her hand, hard, in the meat between thumb and forefinger. A rill of blood spilled out. Then she clawed her cheeks. Although the nails had been clipped back to the quick, they still split the tanned-hide texture of her cheeks in fine red lines.

By this time the door had burst open, and two strong male nurses came in, with Nurse Patterson's pumps thundering behind them.

'That's it, boys!' Carol said, as they took hold of her arms, and forced her to the floor. 'Any second now! Let's have the good stuff! I'll show you a vein, if you like!'

'Leave,' said Nurse Patterson to Freya and Glenn, her face flushed. 'Right now.'

36

On the path back towards the main gate, Glenn practically danced around Freya.

'Have you ever seen anything like that? She was in control, it seemed. Totally compos mentis. All in order and above board. Then at the end… My God.'

'Is this exciting for you, or something?'

'Yeah! Well… Not regarding her.' Glenn relented a little. 'That was bad news. But we got some stuff out of her. It proves it, doesn't it? Your dad didn't kill June Caton-Bell. This seems beyond doubt, now. The cops covered up what happened!'

'I know that.' Freya shook her head. 'I helped blag our way in, all right? I get that. But what happened in there was my fault. For all we know she's been Tasered or something. People can die in restraint. It's partly my fault.'

'Freya, don't worry about it. You didn't provoke anything in there. You just asked some questions, and you got what sounds like the truth. People would kill for that sort of lead, you know, in our profession. This could be life-changing. For you, me, your dad…'

'This wasn't a path I wanted to follow. That's all. I know

it was my idea. But now we've gotten through that, I'll never do it again.'

Glenn kept quiet, and ground his teeth on the way back down the path towards the main gate. 'Why so glum?' he asked. 'We got something good out of her, didn't we?'

'Got something? Maybe so. But what we did today was morally wrong. The woman was upset. And that's before we take into account her massive mental health problems.'

'She's an attention seeker. Might have had psychosis, diagnosis of mild schizophrenia... But I'd say it's a personality disorder she's got. And one or two of her doctors over the years have agreed. Bad, not mad.'

Freya stopped. 'What makes you say that?'

'I may have seen her medical notes.'

'How, exactly?'

'I told you before... I've got my sources, same as you.'

'I think we went too far with that. I'm stating for the record, this was a bit much.'

Now it was Glenn's turn to look annoyed. He folded his arms, and actually pouted. 'Oh, don't start, Freya. You set it up. You could have raised your very noble protest at any point – could have called it off at the last minute. But you didn't. You wanted to find out something, same as me, and you did. Maybe you can do your agonising when you type up your next think piece for some horrendous right-wing rag.'

'Yeah. I'll leave you to type up your exaggerated man-of-action blog.'

'Exaggerated? What are you talking about?'

'I read it last night. How you "gave a warning shout", and threw yourself forward when I was being pursued by a shadowy figure. Gave me a laugh, I have to admit. I was waiting for you to tell your readers how you carried me to safety in your big strong arms.'

'That's what happened… Listen, you were there. You remember it differently, that's your problem. What do you want, exactly? Star billing? Maybe save that for your articles with Mick Harvie.'

'Yeah, I will.' She sighed. 'Look… I'm sorry. Let's not fight about it. For the record, this wasn't good. It crossed a line. We should be wary of it next time. We're the goodies, aren't we?'

Glenn refused the olive branch, and continued to pout. 'I'll try to be worthy of your high ideals in future.'

'Don't patronise me. You never told me about your girlfriend, though it's obvious enough why you didn't.'

'My girlfriend's none of your business.'

'Well, I slept with you, and she gave me a makeover with a hot and sour seafood soup the other night, so you've kind of made her my business.'

'I think we need to leave this for a while.' He looked on the verge of tears; he had a crumpled aspect, like a derelict building the day before demolition. Freya saw for the first time that he was exhausted.

'Listen,' she said, softly, laying a hand on his shoulder. 'We came here to find something out. My motivation's different to yours. This is for my father. Now, we've just heard that he is weird – on a weird scale of one to ten, he's an eight or a nine. Ten being a serial killer. And even before we found that out, everyone I've spoken to about him has told me that the guy's bad news, and I can believe that. A glib, slippery charmer, who takes what he wants and leaves.

A drifter. A womaniser. I'm proof of that. But I think it's possible that he isn't a murderer. The only evidence that points to him having killed someone is fabricated. We know that, now. You want to attach a noble cause to what we did today – that's it.'

'We're forgetting about the body. He knew it would be there.'

'That's going to plague me. Maybe he found the body, and… I'll have to ask him.' She sighed.

'You know and I know that he didn't kill June Caton-Bell. Now we've got probably the real Woodcutter, playing games with us, and the press, and most importantly the police. I've got a duty here. No matter what we think about my dad, what he got up to in his personal life… He's in jail for something he didn't do. They didn't charge him with the other murders – and they were desperate to. There's nothing to connect him with those. They got him on circumstantial evidence, then got the only person who could have cleared him taken out of the play. Now I've met Bernard Galvin – I was told he was a great policeman and a good bloke, then I watched the same person who praised him getting his face broken by him. I'm prepared to believe that on top of being extremely violent, he's also corrupt to the core. We've got a story here. We're in the middle of the story. So, let's finish it, together. But let's keep it official, if we can. No more corner-cutting. No more blagging, no more changing our stories, like we did near the old mine. We play it as straight as we can.'

Glenn looked relieved at this. 'Agreed.' They shook on it. And continued on towards the main gates. They were buzzed out by a security guard on the high, spiked iron gates.

'How about we grab some lunch?' Freya asked. 'Take stock a bit.'

'That'd be awesome.'

Then they heard an engine revving up. They both stepped back, alarmed, as a car roared towards them. It was a sporty little TVR from another world, with iridescent paintwork that reminded Freya of a fly's eyeball. It screeched to a halt in front of them, and the driver got out from the low door in a tangle of legs and blonde hair.

It was Cheryl Levison – Solomon's lawyer. She was furious, her eyebrows at a ferocious angle like a pair of knitting needles. 'Hold it right there,' she growled. 'Both of you, stop. I want a fucking word.'

37

If Cheryl Levison had looked as if she had been on a dirty stop-out when Freya had first met her, here she looked as if she'd dragged herself off the couch after a long weekend spent watching movies and eating crisps – wine included, perhaps.

She wore no make-up, and while still an undoubtedly striking-looking woman, dark rings circled her eyes, and a patch of dry skin floated on her pale cheek. Compared to how she'd looked before, this Cheryl Levison might have had radiation poisoning.

'Whatever you're doing here,' Levison said, 'or whatever you're *thinking* of doing – stop.'

Glenn was utterly flummoxed. 'Who the fuck is this?' he spluttered, turning to Freya. 'You know who this is?'

'Meet Cheryl Levison,' Freya said, dryly. 'Daddy's lawyer.'

'That's correct. Now, before we get to the question of how you ended up here, and ended up inside the building, I need to ask you: what did Carol Ramirez tell you?'

'None of your business,' Glenn said. 'I don't know who you think you are, but you've no right accosting us on the street and making demands. Get back in your sporty little number and take yourself off to the furthest fuck, love.'

Levison looked as if she might swing for him. Freya wanted to take a step back at the sight of the lawyer's hand muscles and tendons bunching. 'Don't be cheeky, son,' Levison said. 'For your information, I'm representing Carol, as well as Gareth Solomon. And if you publish a word of what she's told you, whatever it was, you're going to screw up the appeal. We are days away from the judgment.'

'I thought that was months away?' Freya asked.

'It's been accelerated. There've been one or two developments in your dad's case. You two have been up to your necks in two of them.'

'Meaning the bodies?' Glenn said. 'Old bodies, or the new one?'

Cheryl Levison did not answer this. Addressing Freya, she said: 'I have been working… flat-out. For years. To try and get your dad out of prison. He did not kill June Caton-Bell. This is well-known, but not established. I've tried to turn this from being a plaything of wet little conspiracy theorists and basement-dwellers like Mr Red Ink, here, into something I can prove in court. And I am so very, very close to doing so. If you put something out into the public domain, you'll fuck the case up. Do not mention anything Carol Ramirez has told you. Got it? You want your dad out of prison, those are my instructions to you.'

'We'll consider it,' Glenn said.

'You'll do it,' Levison answered, glaring at him. 'Or I'll let the police know that you were here under false pretences. Impersonating a relative to get access to a high security unit. That's an offence. Might even get you some jail time. And jail time for an overgrown teenager who still lives with his mum and dad isn't an attractive prospect, is it, Glenn?'

This reference gave Glenn pause; he was on the back foot now. 'This changes nothing,' he stammered. 'Don't lecture us, and you've no right…'

'Shut up,' Levison said, pointing at him. 'You've done some excellent work, credit to you for that. I don't know how you found the bodies or who tipped you off – that's one for the police to sort out – but don't mess up my appeal. Or I'll end you. Got it?'

'That sounds like a threat,' Glenn said.

'You're a clever clogs. I can see why you like him, Freya.'

'How'd you find us?' Freya said.

'Quite simple – I'm Carol's lawyer, as well as your dad's. I asked her to get in touch should anyone try to visit her, while all this is going on – anyone at all. She did it only this morning. I almost missed you. Which would have been a shame.'

'Now you've given us the warning – why don't you do one yourself?' Glenn asked.

'I want to ask a number of questions, in fact. Mostly about how you managed to blag your way into the secure unit.'

'As a lawyer, you'll understand if I tell you absolutely nothing about that,' Freya said.

Cheryl Levison got back into her car. 'Remember, kids – I am deadly serious. Do not publish anything about what Carol Ramirez said. I'm not being cute. Keep quiet, and you'll keep him out of jail. That's what you want, isn't it?'

Freya said nothing.

'I'm sure I'll see you around, some time. Keep your eye on the news.'

The car cleared its throat, turned in the road, then vanished.

'I'm not sure whether things just got better or worse,' Freya said.

Glenn ignored her. He had already fished out his mobile phone, fingers scrolling up and down the screen. He looked ashen. 'God,' he said.

'What is it now?' Freya said.

'It's Jools. She's got in touch.'

'Jools? Your girlfriend?'

'Yeah. I'm sorry, I have to wrap this up. It's been too much… This is too much. Today. The past week. I've let this take over. I've got a life. I'm so sorry, Freya. I need to check out for a bit.' He began to walk down the road, towards the bus stop.

'Wait up… At least let me come with you on the train.'

'I'm sorry, we can't see each other for a while.' He was determined.

'I thought you said it was over?'

'It's complicated. We've got things to sort out.'

'Look, we're in the middle of something big. This could be your entire career…'

'I said, drop it!' he roared. 'This is turning into a joke, it's out of control. I'll be in touch.'

'Please… I need help,' Freya said. 'I don't want to be on my own, with this. There's someone dangerous out there.'

'I said I'm sorry.' He strode away.

38

Hey, there! I'm still here, don't you worry. Don't you worry, lass.

It's a strange old road, this. I always knew things would get weird again at some point. How could they not? There has to be an end point. Hey, that's how I planned it. I knew there had to be a full stop. I just never knew where to drop it. I just didn't know the details. You know this, my darling. You know this is going to happen. A meeting. A reckoning.

If I draw a hand across your cheek, will you flinch? I'll do it now. Just a finger, a delicate trace down to where your jaw meets your neck. That's where I'll hit you. Not at first, but that's the killing stroke. I enjoy that one above all. You'll gush. You won't believe it's happening. With luck you'll get a second or two of awareness, of consciousness, before the curtain comes down. Then I get to go to work on you. Then I get to turn a person into a not-person. An unperson.

So, you won't mind if I speak to you a little before I do that. Before I make you run. Before I come after you.

All you are is pixels at the moment, a face on a screen. But we're going to get together before too much longer, I think. You might even be my last job. Not a bad way to go, I guess.

Big job coming up. I'll need to look lively. And a few loose ends to tie up, no doubt about that. I've been bowled a few strange ones of late, and that's the truth. I've got a few bits and pieces I need to find out about.

Still. Best I get prepared.

An axe needs taking care of. Like any other blade, it can lose its edge. So I'm going to keep your face up there, on the screen, while I make a few sparks. And you'll know its edge for real, soon enough. That's a promise.

39

Freya slept far too late. She struggled awake, well into the morning, flapping at her phone handset. The pale blue glow lit up her features. Then she clicked on her newsfeed.

Still not quite fully awake, Freya gazed at the scrolling text for a second or two. She may have made a sound – squeal more than gasp. Then she got up and stumbled into the lounge, switching on the TV set. She'd fallen asleep too early, the exertions of the past few days catching up with her. The time was about 11.45; this pretty much guaranteed that her body clock would be messed up tomorrow, too.

She moved on to one of the TV news channels, where the strapline graphic at the bottom of the page was in block capitals – that, plus the whooshing sound that accompanies the BREAKING NEWS script, told her all she needed to know.

The anchor was the type of person you only saw at this time of night, or on Christmas Day. She looked a little unsure of herself, and read something on a screen just off-camera.

'We are receiving reports that a body has been found in Ethley Sands, a former seaside resort on the Yorkshire coast. Sources have claimed… and we stress, this is not the official line… that this does bear the hallmarks of the Woodcutter case, which has of course seen multiple developments in the past few days.'

A selfie image appeared on the screen: a girl with a pink gin in her hand, pulling a ridiculous duck face pout for the camera.

'The family of Esme Vuckovic has been informed. The find comes just days after the body of twenty-two-year-old Alannah McCormick was found near Durden Water. We should of course stress that there is no suggestion at present that these cases are connected to that of the so-called Woodcutter killings, which has seen two bodies discovered dating back to the mid-1990s, although police are keen to stress...'

She texted Glenn. He called her soon after.

'Have you seen the news?' she said.

He answered with a sigh. 'Guess so. Have the police been in contact?'

'No... why would they be?'

'For protection. That's two new bodies, now, people snatched off the street, or out running. If this is the original Woodcutter, or a copycat, he'll be after you, next. The first girl they found at the resort was your age, I think. Fitness fanatic.'

'Have you guys heard anything through your usual channels?'

'No details. No one's sure, but the thinking is that the MO for the original five killings and this one are much the same.'

'It's the original killer,' Freya said. 'I'm sure of it. Maybe he's got a taste for it again. Who knows?'

'The lawyer knew about this,' Glenn said. 'Levison. She

was being coy about it, but she knew, all right. Surely your father must be released? Unless it's a copycat, of course.'

'Copycat? What're the odds?'

'Slightly better than it being the same man, by my reckoning. I'll keep an open mind.' His voice seemed to come through a filter.

'Are you all right, Glenn? You sound... distant. Is everything OK?'

'Sure,' he sneered. 'Why wouldn't it be? It's only my life in tatters.'

'Whatever's going on – don't go through it alone. I'm here. All right? Don't hesitate. Get in touch.'

'Quite needy, aren't you?'

'What?'

'Never mind. I found something else out. I was thinking about our "Two Ways" conundrum. I think I might have solved it. I know where we're going.'

'You're serious? Spit it out.'

'I'm afraid I'm going to have to get cute with you. I'm going to give you a rendezvous point, and we'll progress from there.'

'OK... But why not tell me?'

'I can't be one hundred per cent sure you're not under surveillance. If I was the police, I'd be watching your house very, very closely.'

'I would guess that. That's why I can sleep at night. He'd be utterly insane to try and get me here. But then I guess... he is utterly insane. So, where am I meeting you?'

Glenn told her. 'Might be an idea to bring a heavier coat. Weather's expected to turn. And bring some waterproofs and base layers.'

'Not going on an Arctic expedition, are we?'

'No, but we might get soggy. You're a fitnessy person – you'll have the stuff.'

After Freya hung up, she looked up the location she'd been given – a pub called the Winston Churchill, of all things, with the classic morose bulldog painting image on the sign outside. Nothing about it suggested 'two ways'.

'What's next?' Freya whispered. She was no longer sleepy, her thoughts racing. 'What have you got in store now? What are you trying to do to me?'

40

It shouldn't have been a cause for fear. 'A boat?' Freya asked.

Glenn drew Freya a look that she would not ordinarily have tolerated. 'We were due to set sail about ten minutes ago. Let's get started.'

'You know boats? I didn't know you knew boats.'

'There's lots of things you don't know.'

'Is it yours, or did you hire it?'

'Hired it… does it matter?'

It was called the *Bessie Bow*, a canal barge. It was tied up at the back of the Winston Churchill, a long green and white craft with pretty floral arrangements along its length. The green-framed portholes were lit up with a cosy glow inside.

Glenn reached over to help Freya on board; there was no gangway, and the boat lurched as she stepped aboard.

'What's the significance of the Two Ways, then – you going to tell me or should I guess?' Freya asked, taking a second or two for her balance to align itself with the shifting horizon.

'No, you're not supposed to guess.' That raised his hackles, though. He frowned at her. 'And what's your problem?'

'Not a problem, exactly. Just that you keep making these incredible deductions and leaps of logic.' She folded her arms, defensively. 'It's amazing how we keep hitting the target like this, isn't it?'

'I wouldn't lay claim to amazing, just accurate. Would you rather I got it wrong a few times? Few blind alleys, few false turns? Would that be easier for you?'

'Don't be sarcastic. Take me through your bloody thought processes. Treat me as if I'm not stupid, for two minutes!'

'You suspect me, don't you?' He said it softly. There was something in that tone that caused a jolt of fear. She had a fleeting notion of jumping over the side. At least it was an option.

'Talk me through it, is what I'm saying.'

'OK.' He rubbed at his forehead; she could tell he was suppressing anger, and she chose not to probe further. 'It took a bit of fuzzy logic – and we could be way off course. There's a place further down called the One Of Two. It's a fork in this canal route. Something about it rang a bell – plus, this place is quite remote, considering it's part of a major canal network. Used to be an industrial zone, donkey's years ago. They keep trying to clean it up every twenty or thirty years, but it always gets overgrown and underused, apart from people on boats like this.'

'In other words, the perfect spot for the killer?'

'Exactly.'

They were in a dark, forbidding place, even at dusk after a warm day. The back of the pub was choked with refuse, obviously during a re-fit, going by the skips out at the back piled with masonry and wooden panelling. There was a quayside here, and one or two empty boats were tied up there. One of them, a crumbling mess of ancient brown paint the colour of dried blood, was named *Zion*. It was an actual sailing vessel with a mast, but no sails, registered in 1922. In the window was a penalty notice of some kind, a modern acid-yellow intrusion. There were net curtains in the windows, but, like the other boats aside from the *Bessie Bow*, clearly nobody home.

'I know what you might be thinking,' Glenn said, as Freya stared at the *Zion*. 'I've already checked it. There's no one on board. No one's been on board that boat for about a decade, I'd say.'

Soon they were untied, and Glenn started the engine. The long finger of the boat edged away from the quay, pointing at an angle into the dark water. The strong bluish light from the fore lights cast a milky light on the waters, startling the leaves green again.

Glenn steered the barge, untying them from the quay, a steady presence at the tiller. Though they were near some fairly large urban developments, close enough to hear the traffic's snuffle and growl, there was a sense they might have been heading into the jungle.

'It was only when I started coming at it from more of an oblique angle that I got some more interesting results,' Glenn said. 'Instead of Two Ways, I looked for One Way Or Another, One Of Two. Six Of One, Half A Dozen Of The Other, that kind of thing. A fork in the road was an obvious starting point. The most interesting hit was One Of Two – and it referred to a fork in the canal network. A couple of miles away. One of the paths takes us down to a weir. It's tough to get there on foot without getting wet, and there's no road nearby. Perfect spot, in other words.'

Freya shivered. 'I wonder if we should have told the police what our thinking is. Tamm did warn us not to get cute.'

'This could be a total wild goose chase. If we call Tamm and he rolls out the complete police experience, and it turns out we've hit a dead end, he'll be angrier than he would be if two concerned citizens called in a body. Or whatever it is we're going to find.'

Freya shook her head. 'I don't get this, Glenn. And to be honest – I don't get you.'

'What do you mean now?' He was exasperated, now, and weary. *Did our relationship just jump forward a couple of years?*

'I mean this is a bit of an about-face. For some reason you don't want anyone to know where we are. Now that there's a maniac out there, I'm thinking we should play it more by the book. He could be out here with us, right now. Waiting for us. The game might be up. We shouldn't be playing at it, any more.'

And he could be right here on deck, with me. All along, Glenn had been a few jumps ahead of her. Putting together the clues, presenting them to her. Pleased with himself – and slightly resentful over Freya's input, whenever she'd been more on the money.

And don't forget, a more feral part of her said, *the guy's a cheat and a liar. Didn't think to mention his girlfriend. On the verge of splitting up? 'Oh, she doesn't understand me; my needs aren't being met'? That's what they all say. And you threw yourself at him.*

'I thought I was following your lead,' Glenn replied, solemnly. 'You've come to me with these clues, remember

– left by some mystery person. Who knows who you are, where you live. Who leaves these amazing clues for you to discover. You must admit, that's kinda convenient.' He raised a hand to cut off her protest. 'I'm telling you how it looks, and how any reasonable person would see it. Definitely how the police would see it. Maybe I'm the one who's taking more of a risk, here. You're the one with the direct link to a guy in jail for murder. And who maybe did several more. So before you start squeezing me into the frame, maybe take a look at how you've behaved, and how it looks.'

'I just want to know what's going on, Glenn.'

'I can take you back any time. I'll do it myself. Or maybe – you want this? For all your protests. Maybe you want to get the truth, and get there first. Given the corruption in this case – it stinks of it, somewhere – maybe we're right to. Pass it on to Tamm, you could be throwing the evidence you need down the drain. Maybe there's someone out there doesn't want your dad out of prison. Maybe the person giving you the information isn't the killer at all.'

Freya didn't address his point. She swallowed her indignation. 'Maybe we'll carry on as we are. But it might be time to come in, now. Maybe we've flirted with it enough.'

'It's up to you.' He faced forward, grinding his teeth. Freya took a moment to calm down.

'Only two left,' Freya said at length. 'Anne-Marie Kittrick and Danielle Pearson.'

'Could be anyone, really. Could be a new body. Could be one of the peripheral disappearances that could be linked in the 1980s. Or it could be nothing.' He sniffed.

Freya zipped her waterproof jacket up to her neck, then

noticed Glenn was wearing a battered suede jacket, jeans and boots.

She pointed these out. 'I thought you said we should wear waterproofs?'

'Yeah. I'm driving the boat. You're doing the action and adventure.'

'What? Myself? You haven't even told me where the fuck we're going!' Suddenly the overboard option seemed like less of a mad notion and more like good sense. The night was a threat, now, without a trace of adventure. 'I'm not doing it alone!'

'You're not alone,' said a new voice from the cabin behind her.

41

Cheryl Levison's waterproof jacket wasn't as loud as Freya's, although luminous slashes up the sides and at the cuffs caught the light in brilliant bolts. She had her hood up, and if it hadn't been for the voice, Freya wouldn't have recognised the shadowy features, backlit by the cosy cabin behind her.

She cursed herself for not checking the boat. *Need to switch on a bit more.*

'Welcome aboard,' Levison drawled. 'I hope you don't mind me tagging along?'

'Bit late to ask for permission.'

'I've got some explaining to do… come on in and I'll brew up a tea for us. Glenn, you want one?'

He shook his head, keeping his eyes out in front. Freya couldn't tell if he was just being diligent, or whether he was ashamed. He looked confident enough on the tiller, with the engine drawling away behind him. The churning of the water was a gentle sound as they cruised along, and with the sound Freya was reminded of holidays.

The cabin was gently lit, and fastidiously clean. A bed with white sheets could be seen, heading towards the bow of the boat, with a galley kitchen and two rows of benches.

One of these had a table bolted to the inner hull, and Levison gestured towards this.

'I contacted Glenn after our contretemps the other day,' she said, as they both sat down on either side of the table. 'Interesting lad. Clever, too. Don't tell him I said that, will you? He could be of use to us, eventually. I've got some things brewing. And I hope you don't mind. I made him an offer – well, I guess I'm making you both an offer. Access to Gareth, the first week he's released. Then three more meetings, lasting a day or more.'

Freya felt a burst of anger towards Levison's insufferably bright tone. 'I don't need you to get access to my dad.'

'True. Well, the offer's for Glenn, mainly, so he can write his blogs and take his photos. Probably won't make any money out of it. But you've got bigger fish to fry, Freya.'

'It's depressing how often people keep mentioning money. Truly depressing.' Freya focused on gazing out of the green-ringed porthole, watching spectral tree limbs quivering at the barge's passage. She wondered what it would be like to live on one of these. To effectively move house whenever you wished.

'It's depressing how many people just put their work out there for nothing,' Levison countered. 'You haven't done that – you sold your stuff to the dailies. You know where it's at. For all your moralising. You're a hunter at heart. Don't be ashamed of it.'

'And what are you hunting?'

'The best deal for my client. That's the contract I've entered.'

'And why are you here, tonight? The judgment is being delivered in a matter of days. Shouldn't you be working?'

'I know my brief inside out, and upside down and back to front, too. That's not a problem. The problem is if something new and unexpected bobs up, and gets in the way. That's why I asked Glenn to let me know if something crops up. He was very generous with the information… But held just enough back so that I'd have to come and meet him. In a lot of ways, I'm lucky he's not some crazed copycat.'

'Maybe you're the crazed copycat, Cheryl? Maybe we should be worried about you.'

The lawyer snorted. 'Nah, don't worry. There's not enough clearance to swing an axe in here.'

Despite Levison's jocular tone, Freya shivered, disguising it by scratching the back of her neck. 'I spoke to Dad a couple of days ago. Sometimes he seemed calm; other times he seemed angry. How's he feeling ahead of the court case?'

'Confident, same as me. As he should be.' Levison sipped at her tea. 'He's quite taken with you, you know. This is really unlike him. If I had to attach qualities to Gareth Solomon, "fatherliness" wouldn't be the first one I'd choose.'

'Lucky for me.'

'Yes… And incidentally, you are his daughter. DNA results came in today, in fact. It usually takes longer to get all these things matched up, but… people do me favours, here and there.'

'Did you have a doubt?'

'When it comes to Gareth Solomon, I doubt many things.'

'But not that he's innocent?'

Levison blinked, as if outraged by the question. 'Oh, he's going to walk free. No question about that whatsoever.'

Freya smiled. 'That's a lawyer's answer, if ever I've heard

one. I wonder if you get too used to lying. You forget that other people can sniff it out.'

'That could be an insult,' Levison said, facetiously. 'But maybe not. I can never be sure with you.'

Irritation quickened her pulse. She had to concentrate hard not to fold her arms, like a haughty teenager. 'I'm going to be honest with you here,' she said, calmly. 'I don't like you being here, and I don't like it being sprung on me. I'll have a word with Glenn about this later. But for now, no more secrets. Don't spring any more surprises on me. This was a nightmare to start with, and I get the feeling it's only going to get worse. I don't like this extra random element.'

Levison gazed at her for a moment. 'Freya, I'm not here to muscle in on your little scheme, if that's what you're bothered about.'

'Don't patronise me.'

The lawyer raised a hand. 'Just a minute. I'm here at Glenn's suggestion. And also at your father's. He's growing concerned that you're in danger on his account – immediate danger, at any time. He asked me to make sure I kept an eye on you. Now before you fly off the handle, I know you're a big girl and can handle yourself. But a little extra help is no bad thing, wouldn't you agree?'

Freya turned away for a moment. That familiar, hopeless longing had returned for a second. The treacherous sense of a burden being laid aside; that her father liked and cared for her. A stranger for all that time.

And still a stranger. Even if he hadn't killed anyone, he had still done unspeakable things.

Freya nodded. 'Fair enough. I guess you're here now. Have we got to go far?'

Levison glanced at her watch. 'According to Captain Flint up there, we're just minutes away.'

'Never seen a fork in a canal before,' Freya said. 'I thought they were just long stretches, like motorways.'

'You can get one or two,' Levison replied. 'Depends on the network. The canal's quite broad, here. Very leafy. Not seen too many boats moored this far out.'

'I'm glad. I don't really want to bump into anyone tonight.'

'Want to head out into the front?' Levison set down her cup.

'Sure.'

Up a short flight of steps to the right of the bed, a hatchway opened out into a tiny area set at the bow. Freya and Levison were a pair of wraiths cast in the strong blue light, and they both turned away from the beam. Glenn was a startled, indistinct shadow through the curtain of light. His head bobbed as he spotted them, then he raised a hand.

Freya returned the gesture, then ducked behind the beam of light. *At least I know it really is Glenn*, she thought. She pictured Glenn's body bobbing somewhere in the subsiding wake of the boat; and his hand replaced at the tiller by that of their nemesis.

Freya peered ahead, where the strong headlight picked out broad, flat dark water. The moon had yet to rise, and even though the headlight was strong, Freya wanted to hold on to whatever daylight was left for a little longer. The towpath was quite overgrown here, with willows dipping their heads into the water, obscuring the narrow paths on either side. Even the sounds of the road had disappeared, this far out, to be replaced by a definite sound of rushing water.

'The way Glenn spoke... It seems you had a falling-out,' Levison whispered.

'True enough,' Freya admitted. 'I haven't spoken to him for a little bit. Think he has a few problems back home that he can't get out of.'

'Oh yeah. Girlfriend leave him, or something?'

'In a nutshell. Though he says it's complicated,' she added, dryly.

'Strange one. First glance, I'd never have put him down as a ladykiller. You never can tell, though. What do you think?'

Freya shut this down, straight away. 'What are you going to do if we do find a body out at the weir?'

'First person I'll call is Tamm,' Levison said. 'I'll relish telling him, I can tell you. I think he's a fraud, and not that good a copper. Type of guy who puts on a smiley face and thinks he's clever. It might work if he was a spiritualist. Less of a good look for the police.'

'He seemed sincere.'

'That's exactly what I meant.'

Suddenly, a new beam stabbed out into the night, out to port. Glenn had switched on a torch. A powerful, bluish ray swept either side of the bank, finding only fencing, green leaves, and the odd black roil of tarmac or pitted concrete as the paths came into view.

'What's up?' Freya asked, tempted to duck down. 'See someone?'

'Nah, checking our situation either side,' Glenn called out. 'We're almost there. Got to admit, I'd rather have tried to force our way through on foot rather than do this. We're piggy in the middle, here. Too easy, if someone took a shot.'

'I don't think that's his style.'

'I wouldn't be too sure,' Levison interrupted. 'When the Woodcutter snatches people, he's pretty persuasive. The only way he'd have gotten Max Dilworth to comply with whatever he wanted was to threaten to shoot him. And he'll be good with firearms, too. Good enough to get a fighty, beery, strapping squaddie to play whatever game turns him on.'

'Strange that the Woodcutter got a result, every time.'

Levison frowned. 'How do you mean?'

'You would think at some point, someone would have called his bluff. Especially Max Dilworth. But if he was the skeleton in the field, it looks as if he took his chances and ran. That's something that doesn't quite add up. Unless we find the last two bodies, and they had gunshot wounds, they all ran, it seems.'

'I hadn't thought of that,' Levison said. 'Maybe Max Dilworth makes the most sense. I got access to restricted papers on him, when I was preparing the case. Stuff that Glenn over there didn't even get to see, thanks to his contacts. Dilworth's bleep test was about the best I've ever seen. It was like happy hardcore before he tapped out. He was a stringy guy, like a featherweight boxer, you know that way? All gristle rather than muscle. And he was fucking hard. I read his reports. One of these people you wouldn't want to either race or fight. Brave, too. Clever enough, as far as those boys go. So, whatever it is our man does to get them into the situation, then to go through with it, then actually chop them up… We've got to be so careful. Hey. This is it. Glenn? You see it?'

'I see it,' Glenn said.

The sound of the engine grew deeper, and the leisurely pace slowed to a crawl. A new sound cut over the top – running water, loud, but with no obvious source. It was almost full dark, with a fine smattering of stars starting to appear in the indigo skies above. It would be a fine night with a fire pit and a few beers, Freya thought wistfully.

The fork came up. 'More of an island than a fork, I'd say,' Freya said to Levison. 'Is that just trees growing out the waterline, or is there any land?'

'Land, for sure. Or a mudbank, most likely. Look. I can see an old traffic cone there... And a couple of tyres.' She grinned.

With the boat now slow enough for them to confidently step off onto dry land, if they wished, Glenn trained his torch onto the bank, spilling the light over the trees on the mudbank, as he guided the long boat to port.

The boat continued its momentum, but frustratingly slowly. Freya again felt the need to crouch as the vegetation closed in – once or twice, seemingly close enough for the branches to reach out and clasp her by the neck, if they wanted to – and the canal narrowed.

Freya didn't want to speak.

Then Glenn said: 'There it is. Just up ahead. You see it?'

Looking to port, Freya could see the canal was in quite an elevated position; the lights of a town sparkled in a valley below. Then the bank to the left disappeared behind a concrete buttress, with peeled white-painted fences standing like a row of drunk men. Water rushed through this fencing.

'That'll be the weir,' Freya said. There was something about the peeling paintwork, the naked railings and the latticework of moving shadows that discomfited her. The liminal feeling of a playpark or a schoolyard in the dead of night, cleared of people. There was only dread here.

42

Freya slid her mobile phone into a zip-lock plastic bag, and slipped it into her jacket pocket.

'What if he's waiting there for us?' she mused. 'He was waiting for me and Glenn at the slate mine.'

'It's possible, but unlikely,' Levison said. 'He wasn't waiting for you when you found the first body, in the farmer's field. He wasn't waiting for you in the ghost town… unless Tamm is the killer. So if the Woodcutter shows up, it'll be just to scare us. If Glenn is right, there's something here he wants us to find. Something unpleasant.'

'A body,' Freya whispered. 'Almost certainly a body. Danielle Pearson or Anne-Marie Kittrick.' She saw their faces, the analogue photographs from the 1990s. Flashbulb images. Honest smiles rendered ghastly, grotesque. Given a tone. They had ended their time on earth in terror. They had run, they had panicked, they had pleaded. And they had found no mercy. Only glee, or rage, or unimaginable lust.

'Hard to say which one it might be,' Glenn said, as he tied up the boat at some cleats fastened to the concrete edge of the bank. 'They were both abducted within about a fifty-mile radius of here. That's what drew me to the canal. The other two locations were triangulated with where they went missing, as well as the possible location. The thing that threw me a little bit is that it crosses into a different county, so whenever you read about the disappearances, you mentally process it as two very different locations, in their case. But in terms of physical distance it's not too far at all. You ready?'

Freya tightened the string at the bottom of her waterproof trousers. 'Sure. What's the deal here, do you even know what you're looking for?'

'Yeah. Safest place to stow a body.' Glenn fixed a bulbous torch to a headband, giving him the look of someone who has been controlled by the Daleks.

'Let's do this. I'll guide you through it.'

'What about her?' Freya nodded towards Levison.

'She's looking after the boat. Any trouble, she hits the horn, we come running.'

'What about if we get in trouble?'

'Then you climb fast, or you jump into the lake at the bottom,' Levison said. She made her way back to stern and hopped back on board, scanning her surroundings somewhat uneasily.

'That's another reason you brought her along – extra pair of eyes,' Freya said.

Glenn nodded. 'She has her uses, no doubt about it. A good person to have on the inside, all told.'

The *Bessie Bow* was berthed alongside a walkway that passed over the weir. The drop down the other side of the elevated part of the canal was not especially steep, its man-made concrete stages looking much mellower than the sound would have had Freya believe. To fall off here would not necessarily be fatal, unless she landed on her head. The weir opened out onto another waterway, perpendicular to the canal up above – a broad, dark lake. There were no houses within sight, but there were some very distant street lights up at the hills. It was a dark, lonely spot, and Freya knew in her bones that Glenn had called it correctly.

Glenn stepped off the boat and onto the concrete running alongside. He uncoiled a guide rope from around her shoulder, then fixed a harness to the white railings at the edge of the walkway. He gave Freya a harness, and attached them both to separate ropes, which he coiled down the side. 'We just let ourselves down, now, bit by bit. It's just insurance really – we won't be going down a cliff face, it's a short drop. Not much water, either. Slippery enough, I guess.'

After one last check through with Levison – who maintained her poise, but had taken to chewing gum quicker than a sclerotic football manager, blatant even in the falling darkness – Glenn prepared to drop down onto the first stage of the mini-dam.

He took hold of the rope, and dropped down onto the slick steps – a drop of about four feet. He landed solidly, bending his knees to absorb the shock.

The weir was a set of four stages, stepping down into the dark water down below. Clearly designed to take the extra water. Freya imagined it was necessary for any overflow from the canal above, during bad weather. She remembered one of the old industrial canals where she used to live, and the constant dredging work that went on during prolonged rainfall – great brown scoops in the earth at the canal bank.

Freya took hold of the rope and dropped down onto the

first stony stage. 'I can't see what we're looking for,' she said. 'Just looks like a set of steps. Big ones, all the same.'

'We drop down one more level, then we're at the main ramp. There's a broad pipe, which turns into an aqueduct, stretching across the weir. I think it helps distribute the flow of water. Not sure where it runs off to...'

'So, one down again?' Freya asked.

'Yep. Unless there's something written here, somehow, some message we're meant to follow...'

Glenn played the blue beam of light across the water. Everything was slick, and there was a slight smell of vegetation that was hard to place – not quite a sea smell, and far from the scent of stagnant water, but not pleasant.

'Nothing,' Glenn said. 'OK. Down we go.'

They followed each other down the second stage. This was a much larger drop, eight feet or so, and the sporadic momentum of the water gained force, here. Freya had to imagine what it was like during overflow, with the white caps as the water surged over the stolid black stone and concrete. Glenn dropped down easily, his booted feet making contact with the wall just once, then landing just as easily as before.

'You're not going to like this,' he said, 'but I'm going to explain this really carefully. For Christ's sake, don't let go of the rope. Let it down inch by inch. I don't want to have to call out an air ambulance because you've broken your back out here. Just take it step by step, hand over hand. It's not very far.'

Freya ground her teeth – irritated not only by the schoolmarmish, condescending tone, but also the knowledge that she needed the instruction. She gasped as she turned her back, and gravity clutched her shoulders. She bumped down in a very gauche, slow fashion, and Glenn compounded the humiliation by taking her weight briefly before she got to the bottom, then patting her on the back for her effort.

'What now – split up?' Freya asked, indicating the dark tunnels at either side of the platform, disappearing into the step, overgrown hillsides at either side of the weir.

'Not on your nelly,' Glenn snorted. 'Left or right?'

'Left feels right to me.'

'OK then.' He started forward, picking his way carefully across the broad-stepped platform. Water trickled down from above, and sloshed unseen under their boots.

'If the Woodcutter jumps out at us, here… assuming he gets you first, what should I do to get a hold of Levison?'

'Shout – very loudly. And hope she's clever enough to call the police before she gets brave. But personally speaking, I think she made the right call on the boat. I'd get the harness off, and jump down onto the final stage, then into the water. Swim hard, make the bank, run for your life. You're a runner, right?'

'Quite difficult to get this harness off while a maniac is running at me with an axe.'

Glenn sighed. 'That's the best I've got. Come on, let's do this.'

Freya hesitated, rubbing her hands.

The head torch blinded her for a second. 'What's up?'

'Just… freaking out.' She gave a small, nervous laugh. 'I just realised I never want to see another body again. I…' Her voice caught. Glenn came forward, instinctively, taking her hand. 'I'm not just doing it for my dad. I'm doing it for them. I've gotten to know them, in a way. Been reading about them. I've had nightmares. Some nights I've slept with the lights on, like a kid. I'm telling myself it's the right thing to do. It's a way of getting to the truth. It's a way of bringing those girls home.'

'And catching the guy who did it,' Glenn said, quietly. He still had her hand. She gave it a squeeze.

'Damn right. There's a sicko out there. I think we can stop him.'

'Let's crack on. Yeah?'

She nodded. 'Yeah.'

The head torch beam lit up the tunnel ahead. It was, regrettably, big enough to walk through, if you crouched. Glenn moved forward slowly. The sound of water echoed off the smooth, circular side of the tunnel. Here, there was no doubt that the water had become stagnant, and there was a smell of carrion here, too. As if some birds had died, Freya thought. And then she thought about it some more.

'Hang on,' he said. 'You see this?'

'No.' Freya came forward, and stared over Glenn's shoulder. Just inside the tunnel, the light disappeared. It was difficult to say what was blocking the way; Glenn's beam showed something matted, some sort of black, fibrous material. It didn't block the entire tunnel – it stretched from the roof, until about six inches from the floor of the tunnel. There was a three-quarter eclipse effect, with the top of the tunnel completely blacked out.

'There's metal down there,' Freya said. 'Some kind of trellis, or something?'

'Looks like a sluice gate. A natural barrier.'

'To stop dead things getting in,' Freya muttered. 'What in God's name is that stuff on the top?'

'It's really mouldy, discoloured, and disgusting,' Glenn said, with distaste. 'Some kind of blanket, or a carpet or something. Hard to say. It's black and slimy and probably full of critters.'

'Nice. Take a bite, for a million pounds?'

The head torch beam lit up Freya's face, and she tried to smile through it. 'Not for two million,' Glenn answered, finally. 'This is tricky… I think we should go through.'

'How we going to do that – limbo dance?'

'No,' Glenn said, properly irritated now, 'we pull aside this material or the sluice gate or whatever, and we go through.'

'What if it's bolted?'

'Then, we check the other side, and if it's the same, then we've made a mistake.'

'What if it's something in the lake at the bottom? That's my guess.'

'Then, Freya, you can come back with some scuba gear and take the fucking plunge, can't you? Let's give it a try.'

'Maybe we should stand off the side, a little.'

'Right,' Glenn snarled, 'you stand off to the side, and I'll take the risk!'

'I don't want to set off a trap or something. This fucker is sneaky. I don't think he's trying to kill us, but I can't rule it out, either. I don't know what the endgame is. Especially when we get to the last of the bodies.'

'Let's find out! One… two…' Grimacing, Glenn took hold of the black material, and pulled.

43

'Ugh! Jesus!'

Glenn staggered back, towards the drop to the third level. Freya reached out instinctively and grabbed him; they steadied themselves. Glenn's light ricocheted off the dark, dripping concrete tunnel exposed beneath the sheeting, a frantic fairy light rebounding off all surfaces.

Eventually the beam settled, and Freya saw what had startled Glenn.

It was a skull – grimy, mouldy, and placed on a bed of bricks on top of a rib cage. The lower jaw was missing. Cutting across one eye socket, moving diagonally across the nasal cavities and ending in a gap in the front teeth, there was one single, obvious cut.

'Christ,' Glenn said. 'No prizes for guessing how they got that wound.'

Freya's voice was a croak. She had begun to shiver, uncontrollably. She felt a sense of disgust down to the marrow, at the idea of stepping into this very water. 'They've been cut in half. Look at the spinal column. Down there… that's a pelvis. I hope to God this person wasn't alive when it happened.'

They let this thought wander for a few moments, as the beam traced the contours of the skull.

'Shut it off,' Freya said. 'I don't want to look at it any more.'

'I doubt this has been here for twenty-five years or so, do you?' Glenn said.

'No.' Freya took a step forward, her heart still thumping. She took a quick glance up towards the lip of the weir, up above. Water dripped down; the rope wriggled as Glenn shifted his position. 'The bones would have been moved, surely… and whatever the hell that material was, it's fairly new-looking, to me. I'd say whoever placed the remains here has been here very recently.'

'Look,' Glenn said, moving closer. He pointed past the skull, to the slick darkness behind it. 'Something's written on the wall of the tunnel.'

Freya came forward, grimacing at the close proximity of the skull. She bent forward, shining her light on the curved concrete that fed into the hillside.

Written in black paint, across the curve of the tunnel, was the message: NO HALF MEASURES.

'Bloody comedian,' Glenn said, grimly. 'Not sure I like this guy.'

Their breathing was laboured, echoing out in that cramped space, as they struggled to recover themselves.

'How old is this part of the weir?' Freya asked.

'I don't think this section is even that old. Neither's the sheeting – you're right. It's been done recently, all right. By someone who really knew what they were doing.'

'It's freaking me out,' Freya said. 'It looks like there's a finger bone, in there. Is it… pointing?'

'Not at us.' Glenn nodded in the same direction the nude fingerbones indicated. 'Over at the other end of the drainage pipe. Far side.'

'You're joking.'

'I'll go first.'

He passed in front of Freya, the rope coiling in front of her shoes, a treacherous creature in the wet half-light. Glenn padded over the concrete platform, pausing for a moment to stare down at the drop below. 'Can you feel a bit of a breeze?'

'No. Not that I'm aware of. Why?'

'I think we had a bit of run-off come down, there. Seems a bit wetter, anyway.' He moved on towards the second drainage pipe.

They both edged closer in the darkness. Something that Freya might have sworn was a bat flew overhead, startling her; something wispy and indistinct, like an ember thrown into the breeze.

'I can't see a grille there, either,' Glenn whispered. 'All clear. There's something in the tunnel, though – written on the walls. Can you make it out? My eyesight's pretty good, but…'

She trained the beam on the writing edged into the wall. It was smaller than the writing they'd encountered before. 'Hang on a minute,' Freya said, 'let's have a look… It says TO ME… TO YOU?'

'Not sure,' Glenn replied. 'I'll have to move further inside.'

Freya placed a firm hand on his elbow. 'Don't do that, please.'

'We need to know, don't we? I can just about make it out.

TO ME... TO YOU. You're right. Let's take a look; there might be something further ahead.'

'Are you joking?'

The light shone into Freya's face.

'Do I look as if I'm joking?' he snapped.

'Well you sound like you're joking, sometimes! Is this some sort of dare? A bet you've got with yourself?'

He ignored this, and took a half-step into the dripping tunnel ahead. 'You coming?'

Freya shook her head. 'No,' she said, simply. 'No to everything.'

'You what?'

'Stop what you're doing. No more investigations. I've had enough. It's obvious that there's another body in this tunnel. He's placed the final two bodies down here. Maybe he's in a hurry. That's up to him.'

'We have to check – we have to be sure. You of all people, Freya...'

'It's not our job, Glenn. It's the police's job. We've messed with evidence already – we can talk our way out of that. Or you can. But if we then mess with another body site, that puts us on dodgy ground.'

'I say we should be sure. You want to know, don't you?'

'It'll come out, one way or the other. Or is it just that you want to know? To get the scoop, for your blog?' She gestured in disgust. 'I'm done with it. It's over.'

Glenn lowered his head a moment, the torch beam threading the moving water with pale blue lightning. He considered this a moment, then said: 'Maybe you're right. It's been getting to me... It's definitely been getting to you.'

'It'd get to anyone. We're messing with evil, evil stuff. Maybe it's all over now. I'm kinda glad.'

'What about your dad?'

'That's for the courts to decide, now.'

Glenn nodded towards the channel. 'That's the pair of them, I'd bet. We've found the last two victims. Unless the Woodcutter's sprung a surprise, and this isn't who we think it is. So, what's next?'

Freya said: 'We call Tamm. Like you said. You'll get your shot at him, now. It's game over. Let's get out of this disgusting place.'

'But what about Levison?'

'She can agree, or walk the fucking plank.'

44

Later that evening, more blue lights, fairy garlands for the trees, meandering gas jets on the choppy water.

Tamm handed Freya a coffee. 'No doughnuts, I'm afraid. Something of a cliché. But we do have bad coffee.'

'Yeah, I remember.'

They were stood on the B-road adjoining the canal, behind a cordon that had been set up with commendable speed. Freya had already had a statement taken, and she had pretty much told the truth. She was expecting another long night of questioning, although Tamm had appeared to take everything at face value. The police sometimes know when you're lying, she reminded herself. She still wore the same clothes; she and Levison had thankfully escaped a soaking.

'I don't know where this ends,' Tamm said to her. 'Four bodies have turned up, recently, connected to the old case; now there's two new bodies.'

'Two?' Freya glanced up sharply. 'There's another one?'

'Yeah. Found near a canal bank, Lancashire,' he said, grimly. 'It's hard to know what to make of it. What do *you* make of it?'

'Hard to say,' Freya said. 'Other than it proving my dad's innocence.'

'You're sure about that?'

'Who else could be leaving messages, spray-painting graffiti, and God knows what else?'

'Could be someone connected to your dad. It doesn't mean your dad didn't do it. Could be the same person who killed the two new girls. Might not. I keep an open mind.'

'So do I. But don't argue against the obvious. We know my dad didn't kill the two new girls. That's a fact.'

'We can say that with confidence, yes.' Tamm swirled what was left of his coffee in the cup. In the gloom he was a curious figure. The long hair might have been stylish a long time ago – say, the mid-1990s – but Tamm was far too old for long hair. He'd washed it that day, but not brushed it, and the light of the street lamps on the nearby street gave him a cosy, fluffy appearance, which he surely didn't intend. Freya wanted to put clips in – the sight was driving her mad.

Or mad-ish.

'So,' Freya continued, grimacing at her own coffee, 'it seems an amazing coincidence that a new phantom tells us about the old bodies, at the same times as new ones start dropping.'

'It is. It's another coincidence that you show up, right around the same time this starts. I'm no conspiracy theorist, but you must admit it's odd.'

'It's got nothing to do with me. I found out who my father was, and I went to find him. It's been a weird time.' She looked away for a moment. She was tired, she realised. Go-straight-to-bed, don't-even-bother-with-the-telly tired.

Maybe it was all getting too much. *There's a girl's skull down there, where the troll lives*, she thought. *I saw it. The last person to see her remains, was the person who killed her.*

When she closed her eyes, she could still see it. This was a different kind of death, not the kind she was used to. She'd had enough now.

Tamm's hand touched her forearm, briefly. He withdrew it when Freya looked up, and seemed discomfited for a moment, knowing he'd crossed a line somewhere. 'Freya,' he said, 'there is a real danger now that whoever's out there might come after you. I'm worried about you on your own. I'd love to tell you we could keep an eye on you, but as I said, we're stretched to the limit. Is there a friend you can stay with, a distant relative, anyone?'

She shook her head. 'I'm on my own. I have one living relative that I know of. I don't think he'll let me sleep on his sofa. Although I might be able to, in a day or so.'

'We'll see about that,' Tamm said, tersely. 'In the meantime, please be careful. I'll give you my direct number if you need to talk about anything. If there's any suspicion that anyone is acting strangely near your property, just call, Freya. We're officially worried.'

She nodded, taking his card. 'I'll let you know. That's a promise.'

'When did you put it together?' he said, indicating the place where the police lights strobed.

'About the bodies? This time, I didn't. Glenn and Cheryl Levison seem to have done all the digging. They didn't have anything more to go on over and above what you knew. The message that was sprayed in the cellar basement at the old slate mine. I knew as much as you. I wouldn't suggest they were cleverer than you, of course.'

'Nah, but you would like me to draw that inference. OK. I'll give you that. But you should have called us, let us know. And Levison being involved is just strange. How did she get into it?'

'Long story. She met Glenn, got talking to him. He told her about the clue our friend left. Decided she wanted to be involved. I'm sure there's a conflict of interest, somewhere.' Freya realised for a moment what she was saying – articulating a suspicion that she'd told herself not to reveal. 'But it's all above board. She's slippery, but she's smart.'

'She is that. She seems invested in her client, wouldn't you say?'

'Yeah. As she should be.'

'Please be careful who you trust, and whose confidence you keep, Freya,' he said. 'I've never met your father, but I know all about the Woodcutter case. Whether your dad was the killer or not, there's still someone out there who's connected with this story. They might be killing again, they might be a copycat… who knows? When are you seeing your dad next?'

'I had thought I'd next see him after he's released… But he wants to see me tomorrow, apparently.'

'You're going to the prison again?'

Freya nodded. 'Don't worry. If he says anything incriminating, I'll tell you. If it turns out he is the Woodcutter after all, I'll make sure he stays in prison.'

Tamm's eyes narrowed. 'You have a doubt.'

'Was that a question, or a statement?'

'You seemed certain he wasn't the Woodcutter, before. What makes you doubt him?'

'I'm not sure what to think, any more. Look, it's getting late, I'm tired, and I've told you all I know. Do you need me? Here, sorry?'

A trace of a smile. 'No, you can go. But we'll be in touch. I've got a long night ahead. You take care, Freya. Remember what I said.'

45

'They've found them all? Or rather... you found them all?' Gareth Solomon's reaction was so scandalised that Freya had the queasy feeling he was putting it on.

'I had help,' she said. 'But yeah. Whoever's been leaving clues has been leaving them for me. So I want to ask you, directly – if you know anything about it, you need to tell me. Because I think the Woodcutter might come after me, now.'

'If he does, he'll have me to deal with,' her father said, scowling. 'I'll be out... maybe in a couple of days. It could be that quick. But how could I have anything to do with it?'

'I'm just asking. It doesn't make any sense. There are too many coincidences for it to actually be a coincidence, if that makes sense. I was never much into conspiracy theories, but you could see how someone could apply a bit of twisted logic to what's happening, and how things have happened. Do you know, I read on a message board that people think I'm the copycat?'

'What makes you think it's a copycat? Same guy, same MO, so far as I can see.'

'We don't know that for sure. If you've got a theory, spill it. Who do you think's the Woodcutter?'

Solomon sat back, and pondered a moment. 'What I would be very wary of is some new, damning evidence coming to light, with these bodies. Something that ties me in tight to the new cases. Now that would be an amazing coincidence, wouldn't it? Your conspiracy theory message board weirdos would get their teeth into that, and no mistake. And I wouldn't put it past the police, whether they're from twenty years ago or into the present day. They set me up. It happens. You better believe it.'

'I do believe it. And I agree, it would be another amazing coincidence if they unearthed some new evidence linking you to the murders, just as you're about to be released.'

'That's putting it mildly. I'm expecting it, to be honest. But at least I'll get a little holiday in the meantime, before they find something to charge me with. Hey – you looking forward to court?'

Freya hesitated. 'I don't think I'll be going to court.'

Solomon was dismayed. 'Why not?'

'Because I think I'm finished with all of this. Sorry.' She sighed, and took a moment to compose herself. 'I didn't really think about what I was getting into, here. I guess that's true of most big messes in life. I wasn't thinking straight. I had an idea about what I wanted to do in life... about ten years too late. I never followed it up. I kept all my thoughts and all my ambitions to myself. I wasn't sure I ever had any. Until the day I found out about you. Now I've taken a step into that world... I want out of it. So please. I know you can't say anything to me.' Freya nodded at the guards. 'I know you can't make a big confession, if there's a big confession in you. But I will ask you – it's a question you can answer in your head, and then you can decide how you want to act. OK? I need to ask you, though: if you know who the Woodcutter is, or you have a suspicion about who it is, then get in touch with the police. Use Levison. Use me. Use the governor. Use the big guy, standing at your shoulder there. But please tell someone. Put an end to all this. And when you come out… if you get the result you need… I don't know if we'll see each other, Gareth.'

'Gareth?' He looked genuinely aghast – little faking that, she supposed. 'You said "dad" before. That hasn't changed. I'm still your dad. And I understand how you feel about what's happened. I don't think I'd adjust to the bodies, this world, the one I see in here. It's not natural for anyone. And as far as society knows, I'm a filthy murderer. It's unnatural. So I would agree with you. Just step away.

'As for our relationship… I understand. But try and imagine how you would feel, stuck in this dump, with sickos and perverts, and you hadn't actually done anything. And then you find out that you had something in the world, something no one could take away… and she doesn't want anything to do with you.'

'It's not that I'm rejecting you. It's not that. I'm rejecting this situation. I'll need to step away. Just for a bit. I… I guess I came out of my shell a bit too fast. I see my face in the papers. People want my voice on the telly, on podcasts, on audiobooks, God knows what. And I know now it wasn't for me. It was never for me.'

'So you go back into your shell?' He gave a wry smile. 'I don't think the world is going to work like that. Not for my beautiful girl. You don't have to get used to the world. The world has to get used to you. That's one way to look at it. Being shy is one thing. Being invisible is impossible.'

'You sound like a motivational poster at a gym. That's a big reason I don't go to gyms, incidentally.' Freya pulled a tissue from her purse, and dabbed at her eyes. She frowned at the guard – a new one – when he stepped forward to peer at what she held in her hand.

Solomon raised a hand. 'Not trying to contradict you or belittle what you're saying. Do what you feel is right. And when the time comes, if you feel like getting in touch, having a catch-up, talking on the phone… Do it.'

'What happens when you're released?'

'I get naked and invent cocktails.'

'Apart from that, I mean less important things, like… Where are you going to sleep? Do you have clothes? How are you going to eat?'

'Levison's handling all that, so put it out of your head. Don't worry, I won't be knocking on your door at midnight, demanding a bed, or anything like that. To listen to Levison's plans, a place to sleep of my own won't be a worry. A bit like life in here, now that I think on it.' He tipped a wink to his own guard, who as ever, didn't respond.

'Think you'll move around again?'

'That's a possibility. With a great big pay-off, I might get travelling. It's a big world, and I want to see it. Do you know, I've driven the length of this country, and felt experienced and wise in the world as a result? In actual fact, I just got experienced at parking, and petrol stations. I guess some people get experienced at airports and fancy hotels and expensive luggage. But it's not the same as travelling. Know what I mean?'

'You never really explained that, did you?'

'What? Travelling?'

'Petrol receipts. The ones that link you to the abductions. By a lot of reckoning you drove past every abduction site, at the critical times. Isn't that right?'

'I don't need to explain it. It's all out there, in black and white. As I said – I was a driver by trade. Did long distances. If I was connected to the locations, then so were a lot of other drivers. Coincidence, not causality. And think about it – the petrol receipts. The alleged smoking gun, connecting me to the murders. If I was a multiple murderer, why would I collect receipts that put me in the killing zone? I'd have to be stupid, wouldn't I?'

'A lot of clever people are stupid when it comes to money. Maybe you just weren't thinking straight?'

'It's a coincidence – that's all. It's not a very sexy line to take... You wouldn't read it on a murder blog or a Sunday supplement deep dive into the *mind of a killer*.' For these last words he put on the voice of a horror movie trailer narrator, disturbingly loud. 'But it's the honest, mundane truth. If they'd had any evidence showing I committed those murders, they would have hung them on me in a minute.'

'That's true, it's totally circumstantial. But there's one murder you are connected with. At the moment, it's the one you're guilty of.'

'Well, that's complicated, mainly down to Carol Ramirez.'

'Yes.' Freya closed her eyes; composed herself. 'I spoke to her. She told me about you. What you were into.'

Solomon shrugged. 'Consenting adults.'

'It wasn't normal, though. "Dodgy" hardly covers it.'

Now he looked uncomfortable. 'What's dodgy, really? I'm into women. One of them asks me to put her over my knee, because she likes it, I'll put her over my knee. One of them tells me to put her knickers on, then I hope she's packing strong elastic, because they're on. I've never hidden that. That's what I like. Women. And that's it. I know it's not very interesting. I know it won't sell whatever newspapers still exist. But I'm a meat 'n' two veg kinda person. That's as delicately as I can put it to my daughter.'

'She was on a death trip, wasn't she? Carol Ramirez? And you facilitated it.'

'I was gullible, with hindsight. To be fair, Carol Ramirez? I'd never have forgotten her. It's a shame she was out of her mind. Women like that don't come along too often. Know what I mean, lad?' He grinned at the guard on his shoulder.

The crudity was a deflection, and this irritated Freya. 'But you found the body, didn't you? Then you called Carol Ramirez up, and you spent some time in the woods near the body. Isn't that right?'

'That's not the facts as I understand them.' He blinked when he said it.

'Then tell me the facts as you understand them.'

'Carol Ramirez found the body, not me. That was never revealed in court, because she didn't get near a court. Don't ask me how or why. It did cross my mind she might be the Woodcutter, you know. Carol Ramirez calls me, brings me out to the woods. It turned her on, you see. Death. Being near death. I'm not sure what you'd call it… paraphilia? Something like that? I'm not sure. You'd have to ask her. God forgive me, I went to the woods with her, and we got up to all sorts, but I promise – I didn't know there was a body around.'

'So you were set up – and Carol lied?'

'That's it. I was very unlucky. People believe what they want. They still will, even if I walk in a few days. Another way of looking at it is that I was *lucky* in a way – lack of evidence hasn't always stopped a conviction, in legal history. That applies to me. They could have done me for the lot. I'm lucky they only pinned one on me.'

Freya took a sip of water. 'How long before you finished with my mum, before you hooked up with Carol Ramirez?'

'I'm not sure of the details.'

'You answered that very quickly. Sure you don't want to think about it a bit?'

'That's because I'm not sure of the details.'

'Had you been seeing Carol while you were seeing Mum?'

'It's not impossible. But I don't think so.'

'Lots of women, then, right?'

'Don't be like that.'

'Like what.'

He bit the side of his mouth, then said: 'Look. I'll tell you about Mary Bain, if you want. The Mary you might not know so well. The Mary who existed before you existed. She was beautiful. I remember her, all right. You've kind of got her cheekbones, but not as pronounced. She had the most amazing face. I want to say big-boned, but that sounds like an insult. She was sculpted – could have been a model, easily. Something sad about her. A bit of an enigma. Seemed a little bit like you do now – a bit withdrawn into herself. No real family. Wary of people. The ironic thing being, she drew them to her. Not to say she was man-mad, or anything. When I say she drew people in, she drew everyone in. The older women loved her. Women her own age wanted to be her friend. She listened. And the old boys, my God, you saw some of them losing decades off their lives, when they came in at lunchtime with their dogs. Cologne behind the ears, flowers, even, you name it! She was lovely. What she saw in me… I couldn't tell you, and she obviously didn't tell you, either. We were attracted to each other. We had a summer together. That's all I'll say. A good summer. That's all that needs to be said. Look… I'm sorry.'

Freya was sobbing, now. The guard on her left swallowed, twice, in discomfort. 'It's OK,' she said. 'You've said enough, now. That's the final piece, really. I'll maybe see you after the appeal. I'm sorry, Dad, I've got to go.'

He got up; he protested. She didn't listen.

46

Freya saw Glenn around twenty-four hours later, after she had fought a phalanx of press at her front door. She had taken her bike around the park several times, then took it through the side streets until she was absolutely sure no one was following her. She contacted Levison, asking them to fire a warning shot through the press regulator. The lawyer had already told her in advance that this might prove productive, and certainly couldn't hurt during the furore of the body discoveries.

There was no contact from Mick Harvie.

She had somewhat shame-facedly carried out what she called in her head a 'fact-finding' mission on Glenn, checking out photos on his social media. He'd mentioned a local more than once, an old-man hangout with horse brasses, dark-stained wood panelling and a very basic menu, somewhere he evidently enjoyed drinking alone in a corner alcove. There was a weeknight pub quiz he had gone to several times. The Mason's Mark had seemed the best contender for the pubs around where he lived, and so Freya took a chance.

It was just as it had seemed, even down to the elderly sunburnt red carpet, which, if it was a hairstyle, would have been a combover. It was quite busy, with a pleasingly mixed crowd. She drew some stares as she walked towards the bar, keeping an eye out for any alcoves. There had been several alcoves in the pictures she'd noticed on Glenn's social media.

She saw him beneath a painting of a horse being shod by a hunched, muscle-bound and slightly sinister figure, the shoe glowing with the colour of sunburn in a brazier, the whole scene flecked with sparks. It was rather good, considering. It couldn't quite distract Freya from the scene unfolding below.

Glenn was sat with the girl who had stormed into the restaurant. She stopped, and turned to leave. They both spotted her; the girl got up and walked over to Freya. She had a friendly expression on her face, which Freya didn't trust an inch.

The girl raised her hand. She was dressed in jeans and a smart white woollen sweater. She was pretty, Freya felt, with an odd pang that might have been either envy or shame, with high cheekbones, honey-coloured hair and eyes as blue as Freya's were dark, but almond-shaped, and comely.

Glenn didn't get up, try to stop her, or do anything. He sat, seemingly frozen. Freya thought he might have been dead, in some ghastly twist, until he ran a hand through his hair. He looked exhausted.

'You've sorted out your highlights, I see,' the girl said, not in any aggressive way. 'The brighter colour really suits you. And your face. Although, you know what they say about people who change their hairstyle all the time, don't you?'

This nettled Freya, and she let it show. 'Oh look, save it. I came to speak to Glenn. I'm not interested in your domestic dramas. If you've got something you want to say to me, say it now. I don't have the time or the patience.'

'There's no need to be unpleasant,' the girl said, in the same tone. 'No dramas, like you said. And you're not interrupting anything. You're kind of a full stop, in fact. Glenn was here on his own. I came to hand back his keys. That's done now.'

'Look… I just want to say, I didn't even know you existed until I saw you at that restaurant. I wouldn't dream…'

Now the other grew dismissive, even haughty. 'You're all decency. I can see why he likes you. Anyway – I'll just say this. Glenn isn't into relationships, or into people, particularly. It took me two and a half years to realise that. Maybe you'll realise sooner? Any road up – good luck. Oh, just one thing.'

Freya stood her ground. A nerve jumped somewhere between her ear and her throat; she fully expected the attack to come on the instant. Briefly, her eyes flickered to nearby tables. There was an empty glass. Even better, at her elbow, a bottle which one customer had just put on the table. 'Spit it out, love.'

'If you're a serial killer's daughter, do you think the same things as him?'

Freya blinked. 'I'm not a serial killer's daughter.'

'By that I mean, do you get any mad urges? Any dark thoughts? Think you could kill someone? Good chance it's in the wiring.'

'To tell you the truth, it's crossed my mind once or twice. In the past minute or two.'

'Yeah. Listen.' And then she leaned in – too close.

'You be careful,' Freya said, quietly, expecting the blow from any angle. 'Extremely careful.'

But the stress leached out of the other girl's face, and tears formed in the corners of her eyes, as she said: 'Don't be hurting him. All right? I don't love him any more, but I don't want to see him hurt, either.'

Freya let her pass. Nothing further was ventured. Her back and shoulders still pulled taut with tension, Freya pulled out the chair where the girl had sat moments before. Her hands quivered uncontrollably. She made no effort to cover it, nor the tears that escaped down her cheek. 'So, Glenn,' she said, brightly. 'Busy few days?'

He said, at last: 'Lively.'

'We didn't get arrested. I suppose that's something.'

'Ace.'

'Look. Maybe we should go. This is awkward. Mainly because I don't like sitting here with my back to the door. I'm not sure whether that girl's going to run back in here with a machine gun any second.'

'Wouldn't put it past her,' he said.

She touched his arm. 'I'm not sure if I've said it before… I'm sorry. I feel like I've caused this. If I'd known about her, I would never have…'

But is that true?

'No,' Glenn said. 'I didn't tell you about her. So it's not your fault. I could have stopped it any time. I suppose I… I didn't want to.'

'Oh.'

'Anyway. There it is. She's gone. She's given back the keys. She's taken away all the shit CDs.'

'People still listen to CDs?'

'Some people even listen to vinyl discs on their gramophones.' For a second, he looked as if he might cry; as if he might crumple against her. Freya braced herself for it, the same way she'd braced for Glenn's ex to take a swing at her.

Then he buttoned it up, and sat up straight. 'So. Drinks! You and me. Success. You should see the hit-count on the blog. A couple of the true crime podcasts were in touch.'

'Were the police in touch?'

'Only all day.'

'Me too.' She sighed.

'Get anything out of you?' He grinned. 'That was a joke.'

'I don't think so. Main thing I got out of it… I think they were embarrassed.'

Glenn smirked. 'Because we used a bit of brain power, and found out something at the drop of a hat, and they didn't?'

'Exactly.'

'Makes you wonder whether or not it's deliberate.'

'What – that they're deliberately shit at their jobs?'

'Suspiciously shit at their jobs, might be a better way of putting it.'

Freya lowered her voice. 'Do you reckon the Woodcutter's in the police?'

'When murderers vanish into thin air, and particularly when someone is put away for it in dodgy circumstances, that's when I start to wonder. Hey, I'm thirsty – drink?'

Freya shrugged. 'Why not? I'll take whatever fizzy pop they have on tap. By that I mean, standard-issue lager.'

When he came back, he said: 'They do a quiz on in here later.'

'Yeah, I know. Cheers.' She took a sip. 'You look thin. When was the last time you ate?'

'I dunno. Porridge this morning? Fills me up.'

'Maybe we could grab some nachos or something. Or we could go for a curry?'

'Yeah… I've got some things to work out first, you know?'

'Oh, got you. Legal stuff with your flat, maybe? You having to buy her out?'

Glenn frowned. 'What? No, we were renting. Christ. How much money do you think I have? Nah, I meant, on the case. I've been busy in the background… You look surprised.'

'Yeah, it's just… I thought you might have had some more on your mind, that's all.'

'In what way?' Glenn seemed genuinely puzzled. 'I've got reams of good stuff, you know. I was digging out a few things about the two bodies they found. Some of my people on the ground with the forensics department, they're really good off-the-record. They've maybe seen a bit too much *Silent Witness*, you know?'

'Glenn, I don't want you to take this the wrong way, but… I was thinking you were onto some kind of nervous breakdown because you were breaking up with your girlfriend. Not because you were working overtime on the Woodcutter.'

'We're on the scent, though,' he said, and a strange look took over his face, then – blank, but intense at the same time. He focused on something over Freya's shoulder, something that probably wasn't there, although she did check, just in case his ex was poised to crash a fire axe into her head. 'It's close, isn't it?' he whispered. 'I think there's some sort of breakthrough to come. I'm sure of it.'

'Whatever you say. I'm not sure what's next, though. And I'm not sure I can stomach any more bodies. All four of the missing from the first case have been found. Plus two more that happened recently. Is there an endgame to this? What's his plan? And what's ours?'

'I think he's going to let events churn on,' Glenn said. 'Things are ramping up, now. Especially when it comes to what's going to happen tomorrow.'

'And what's that then?'

'You serious?'

Freya gulped down the pint. 'What have you heard now?'

'She didn't contact you?'

'Who?'

Glenn raised his phone and fiddled with it for a moment or two. 'Here. Look.'

There was a single text message on the screen, from Cheryl Levison. It said: 'Tomorrow. Supreme Court. Judges making their ruling. Get ready.'

Freya said nothing, for a moment. 'No. She didn't contact me.'

Glenn lifted his empty pint glass. 'Another?'

47

Freya watched him sleeping for a good while. She thought he'd been talking in his sleep – something had woken her up, at any rate. But Glenn only sniffled and whimpered a little, his lips moving sometimes, but making no sound. Freya lay on her side in the gloom, focused only on breathing.

She'd decided to stay over; he'd even helped her bring her bike into the hallway, though he had sounded angry when she left a scuffed tread-mark on his wall with her back tyre. All around the flat there were clear spots and blank spaces where a relationship had been erased; even down to squares on the wall where picture frames had recently hung. CD towers were depleted, but not by much. Perhaps the most telling sign was the single dish laid in the drainer in the kitchen, with a knife and fork poking out of a cutlery rack.

They had a nightcap. They'd talked about how weird it would be to do anything daft, and she'd agreed, though she had also suggested bunking up beside him in the bed rather than being huddled on his couch with towels and empty covers. Then of course they'd done it.

Freya smiled in the dark, remembering how he'd gone under the covers in order to take off his underpants – a totally tropical shade of aquamarine, which had almost caused a fatal case of the giggles that could have changed the course of the evening had she allowed them to escape. He'd allowed them to drop onto the floor, agonisingly, from his big toe. That's when she'd gripped the quilt cover and tore it off him.

When she emerged from the reverie, she realised his eyes had opened and he was staring back at her.

'What?' she said, at last. 'Come on, speak. Have you died or something?'

'Just thinking,' he said. He lifted his watch from the bedside table, and grimaced. 'Hours to go.'

'Until what?'

'Court proceedings.'

'Guess we better kill some time, then.'

She reached for him, and his eyes sparkled above his true, unguarded, sly smile.

Porridge for breakfast, sweetened with blueberries and a swirl of honey. They sat in his front room watching a rolling news channel.

'*Stay tuned*,' Cheryl Levison had told Glenn, at about 9am.

Freya licked her spoon, as she considered Glenn's phone screen. 'Going to confess to some jealousy here. Just a little bit.'

'Because Cheryl Levison texted me, and not you?'

'Yeah. Exactly. I saw her first. And he's my dad. What's she doing texting you, anyway?'

'I've been in contact with her for the past ten days or more,' Glenn said, after a pause.

'Even before she stalked us? When we went to see Carol Ramirez?'

'Well… Yeah.'

She gazed at him. 'Want to talk me through your reasoning, there?'

'I was curious. I wanted to see if I could get anything from her. I also think your dad should be free. Cheryl Levison is the one to do it. The link was clear.'

'Did she say anything about me?'

'She said, "I can't figure Freya out. Sometimes she seems to be a smart kid, sometimes dense. The first time I met her she looked like she'd have run a mile if I'd clapped my hands suddenly."'

Freya was actually rattled by this. 'Did she say that?'

''Fraid so.'

'Anyway. I guess we're going to be talking to her quite soon. Something's happening.' Freya indicated the screen, where black and yellow tickertape flashed up, and a superannuated though undoubtedly handsome newscaster frowned as he read it.

'News just coming in from the PA news agency from the Supreme Court, where it's been revealed that Gareth Solomon, the man dubbed the Woodcutter, has been freed on appeal. Three supreme court judges delivered a unanimous ruling that his conviction for the murder of June Caton-Bell was unsafe. Of course, the case was expedited thanks to the discovery of several bodies in the past few weeks, which investigators believe may have been the missing victims of the serial killer known as the Woodcutter. And of course, other bodies have been discovered, subsequent to Gareth Solomon's imprisonment.'

'He's out.' Glenn slammed a fist into his palm. 'He's out! You did it. He's *free.*'

'That's... That's something,' Freya said.

'At least look happy about it! Hey...' Glenn motioned to hug her; halfway through it, he chickened out, and offered a high five, which she reluctantly accepted. 'Is everything all right?'

Freya nodded. 'Just thought about someone.'

'Who?'

'My mum. She was forgotten, my mum. Maybe even by me. Been gone... a matter of weeks. I've still to have my first Christmas without her. No one will think about her. They'll only ever think of me in terms of him.'

'Hey...' Glenn got up, taking care to put down his porridge bowl, and sat beside her. He laid an arm across her back, and hugged her. They sat, awkwardly, perched on his sofa, while a whooshing sound signalled a change of shot as live pictures came in from the steps of the court.

'We go now live to the scene outside court, where Gareth Solomon has appeared with his barrister, Cheryl Levison...'

The image wavered as the cameraman was jostled. His colleagues flashed into view – an unsettling battery of video equipment and camera lenses – before several figures emerged from the court.

One was Cheryl Levison. Freya had to admit she looked amazing, lithe and blonde, chiselled but not hard-looking, like a fitness instructor whose classes you looked forward to. It was only when the man who stood beside her emerged and came down the steps to join her that the strobe light barrage began.

Gareth Solomon wore a metallic blue suit that looked good on him. He looked thinner in normal clothes than he had in bulky prison clobber, and his beard had been removed, leaving a broad, but pleasant face. He no longer had that satyr-like appearance, shorn of his beard, and his dark eyes seemed almost benevolent as he stood on the steps beside Levison. Two minders stood on either side of the pair, both in their late forties or fifties, both wearing outlandishly large coats that made them look as if their hands and faces had been added as afterthought. 'Hard-looking' was a complete understatement.

Levison spoke first, without notes, exultant and confident. 'On behalf of my client I'd like to thank the Supreme Court justices for fast-tracking this appeal, and for reaching the only sensible conclusion: that Gareth Solomon is not the serial killer known as the Woodcutter. He was not responsible for the death of June Caton-Bell, and he was not responsible for the deaths of the other four people whose bodies have been recovered in recent weeks. In our view, the discovery of two more bodies, bearing all the hallmarks of the previous Woodcutter case, rendered the jury's original decision in my client's trial a quarter of a century ago, utterly redundant.

'This has been a grave miscarriage of justice, and once my client has become acclimatised to the freedom so cruelly denied to him all these years, we intend to pursue the matter further. A public inquiry should be established to look at what went wrong.'

'She's good,' Glenn said, absently. 'Can see her in

parliament. Or doing karaoke. One of these really boring bastards who's excellent at it.'

'Furthermore,' Levison said, 'we want to pay tribute to the people who have never given up – who have fought for my client even after he was accused of the most despicable crimes. This country has a tradition of fairness that transcends the ideals of one or two individuals who would seek to subvert it. Our gratitude goes to you.

'And of course, I could not talk about this case without mentioning the five – possibly seven, possibly even more – victims of a sadistic, vicious killer, who is still to be caught. My client is fully aware that even though this is a positive day for him, it means that the suffering, the hurt, the fear and the uncertainty continues in tandem with the grief. Our fight for justice is a fight for justice for the victims, too. Perhaps now, the police can concentrate on lines of inquiry that will lead them to the Woodcutter – the real killer we believe is still active today. That is all. Thank you.'

She stepped back, and there was a cacophonous volley of questions. Solomon looked diffident for a moment, then he gazed coolly at the cameras, squaring his shoulders. He nodded, and appealed for quiet, raising his hand. At this gesture, there was an even greater frequency of clicks and flashes.

'Proper press pack, this,' Glenn said. 'Your dad's big news.'

'All the better,' Freya muttered.

'We should have been there, really.'

'To do what? Get shoved by horrible old men? No, I think we're better off out of it.'

'Might be nice to meet him.'

'You'll get your chance.'

'Seriously?' The hope in his voice irritated her. She did not answer.

In a deeper voice than Freya remembered, her father said: 'I would like to echo what my fantastic lawyer, Cheryl Levison, said earlier. The past twenty-five years have been one long nightmare, and I would say that it isn't over yet by a long way. I have to come to terms with the fact that a significant portion of my life has been destroyed by the actions of corrupt police officers who simply wanted to fit someone up for a series of crimes they could not solve.

'I am not the Woodcutter. I did not kill any of those people, and I certainly was not responsible for June Caton-Bell's death. My thoughts are with the families. I've tried to correspond with all of them. None of them wanted to speak to me, and that is understandable. But I want to say to them – I want the Woodcutter caught. I will launch a campaign, I will do whatever I can, to put this evil man behind bars. And I would say to him now—' here, Solomon gazed right into the camera '—your time is coming. Justice will prevail.

'There are many unsung heroes. One of them is my daughter, Freya, whose work behind the scenes will go down in legend. I don't know Freya as well as I'd like to, but I am looking forward to having a normal relationship with her when the time is right. She has been a tower of strength, and she's only one of many people who believed me, who saw through the lies, who helped me get to this point today. Thank you.'

The anchor spoke over the retreating figures, as the minders closed in, allowing them passage through the cameramen and photographers.

'When you meeting him?' Glenn asked.

'I don't know. I'll get in touch with Levison – assuming she doesn't prefer talking to you. Then we'll meet up. Don't worry,' she added, tetchily, 'we'll find a spot for you.'

48

She didn't, though.

The dimensions of the restaurant changed dramatically once Freya opened the door. Glass doors gave way to a tunnel in stark white tiling, and a roof that got larger and larger as the end of the corridor seemed to get further and further away. Voices echoed from the far end, and the effect reminded Freya of being at a swimming pool. She was glad to reach the reception, then to be shown through a set of heavy doors into the blast of noise that was a restaurant in full swing on a Friday night.

She spotted them quite quickly. It was an effort to control her face.

He was wearing the same odd blue suit she'd seem him on the television a few days previously – she couldn't quite decide what colour best described it. Gunmetal grey or blue didn't quite fit, nor did metallic. It was probably best suited to that slightly iridescent hue of an exotic dragonfly, a shade that caught the eye without offending it. He had a glass of wine in front of him, and was in a state of some merriment. She hoped he wasn't drunk, with what felt like a reflex reaction to a father she'd never known.

Next to him was Cheryl Levison. She wore a pure white

dress, which would have been an invitation for every corpuscle of red wine or red sauce to attach itself, had it been worn by Freya – but she had an inkling Levison might hang that dress back up as pristine as the day she bought it. It was cut deep on her chest, but linked across the collar by a delicate gold chain. She was stunning, there was no other word for it, and her hair had been styled recently, cascades of gold that reminded Freya, ludicrously, of a longed-for pony toy she had asked Santa for, but never received. Every inch of her took effort. She was simultaneously hard to focus on for too long, but impossible to ignore. '*I can see her in parliament*,' she recalled Glenn saying. As euphemisms went, it was hard to beat.

Another man was with them, with a high, receding hairline, glasses and a tweed jacket. He had a pinkish hue to his face, as if he'd recently shed his skin. Freya could only categorise his appearance as that of a teacher who frightened you.

Whatever joke they'd all shared, Freya's arrival amplified the sense of merriment. All three got to their feet. Levison came first, gripping her by the hand and then the free arm. The gesture was proprietorial, but Freya allowed it.

'Freya. God, you look wonderful! Doesn't she look wonderful, Dad?'

'Dad?' Freya said.

'Figure of speech,' Levison said, without breaking stride. 'Hey, would you look at this gorgeous girl, Gareth?'

He took her in his arms without hesitation. 'My girl,' he whispered at her ear. 'My beautiful girl. What a gift. After all this time.'

She laid her head against his chest. She felt a bubble grow

within her, a sensation that was not entirely pleasant; Freya felt as if something must burst inside, that she might emit a sob or a whimper, things she did not want to happen. 'Well done,' was all she could say, into his thick chest and shoulders. 'Well done, you.'

Freya was amazed to see tears in his eyes as he drew back. 'You were denied to me. Of all the things that were stripped away, that's the worst. It's not being locked up. It's the lack of you, in my life. All those moments a dad should share… Christmas…'

'Dad,' was all she could say. The world grew blurry.

The little man in the tweed coat clasped his hands. 'My goodness, darling. What a moment! What a moment!'

Freya turned towards him, rubbing away the tears that dampened her cheek. 'Sorry, who are you?'

'My name is Just Leaving. Only kidding. Here, I won't intrude on this any more, I just can't. But I'll leave you my card. Your dad and, well, Cheryl can fill you in. We'll talk soon, I know it. We'll do great things. I guarantee you.'

He got to his feet with startling speed, tapped Freya on the shoulder and held out a card for her to take. Set among an arresting domino pattern, the script along a white bar in the centre read: William Blessed, Literary Agent. Even as Freya looked up, he was already heading towards the doors.

'He's not hungry I guess,' she said, dropping the card into her pocket.

At the table, her father pulled out a chair, in between himself and Levison. 'C'mon, sit down. We've got lots to talk about. Hope you're not hungry, either,' he said, under his breath. 'Looks like pretendy-food they serve in here. With none of the trimmings.'

A waiter came over to take Solomon's place, and helped push her seat in. A menu appeared in her hand not long afterwards.

'You've got no idea what a novelty all this is,' Solomon said. She noticed he was sweating a little. 'Not that I ever did this too much back in the day. Heh!'

'Glass of wine, Freya?' Levison brought the bottle over and tipped a burgundy measure in, without waiting for affirmation. 'Best of stuff. It's all on me – order what you like. Fillet steak. I believe they do turbot as well – worth having. That's a fleshy fish.'

'Do they do fish and chips?'

'If you ask, they'll probably do it. Or ask you to leave, one of the two.'

Freya took a sip of the wine, glancing around at the other tables. There were suits and fancy dresses everywhere. Freya had opted for black dress trousers she had worn during a stint at a casino eighteen months ago, which mercifully still fit; her blouse over the top was loose and flowery, not her favourite, but her most expensive and unstained top. She had opted for flats after an agony of indecision, but had regretted it the moment Levison had towered over her. The lighting was perfect, as was the seating, allowing for a little privacy among pools of light on the circular tables. The design feature of the restaurant was to remove any and all sharp edges, particularly on a gantry-way that separated the lower floor from an upper tier of seating. It was unmistakeably stylish, but in some places it made the décor look unfinished.

No one appeared to realise who the thick-set, jolly-looking man in their midst was.

'You're looking well,' Freya said to him now. 'I mean, what's the deal – they basically let you out?'

'Yep,' he said, cheerily. He had wider nostrils than her – something she hadn't inherited. They flared, comically, as he took in the bouquet, the tip of his nose inches from the surface. 'Once you're free to go, you're free to go. I'll get a nice parcel of books and whatever from the jail. But that's it. And I'm never going back.'

'What a feeling,' Freya said.

'Don't I know it. You know what they call it – culture shock? Like that?' He glanced at Levison, who nodded, eyes narrowed behind her glass. 'Mobile phones, computers… I knew about these things, but I didn't know how widespread they were. Everything's piped right into your eyes and ears – the news, your music… even your friends' faces. Or a mockery of them. When I first went to jail, a computer was a green screen about the size of this table. You could defrost a turkey on top of it in half an hour. Now they fit in your hand. Now it's all headphones and wireless and God knows what else. Amazing. Like space movies, back in the day. They had an internet when I got locked up, but it was pretty basic. There weren't even pictures. It was all restricted. Now, my God… If you'd told me that the technology was wired right into people's minds, I'd believe you. But listen… there's a whole world to talk about. And I'm so glad I get to talk about it with you.'

'How about literary agents?' Freya asked. 'Were they around, back in the day?'

'Mr Blessed is one of the most renowned literary agents in the country,' Levison said. 'The next time you see him, you should probably genuflect.'

'And I take it he had some good news for you?'

'Yeah,' Solomon said, leaning forward. 'And for you. If you want.'

'How's that?'

'You can write your story,' Levison cut in. 'In tandem with your dad's. Your search for your father. Discovering the bodies. Exonerating him – or, helping to. And then the relationship you've cultivated. Think about it. It's a great story, you have to admit. An innocent man, framed for a murder he didn't commit. And then the daughter he never met, helping him regain his freedom. It's got everything. An amazing story.'

'You want my story? For sure?'

'Yeah, absolutely.'

Levison laid a hand on Freya's arm. 'We are talking, "not having to worry about anything ever again" money. You up for it?'

'I suppose.'

Levison frowned. 'You look like you have a doubt?'

'Well… I'm not interested in money. I've said it before. Mr… what was it again, Blessed? I've had contact from people from his world before. They've read my articles. There's a lot of interest, you know that. It's just… I think I'll tell the story my own way. A book, I mean, I just don't know…'

If Levison was discomfited in any way by this revelation, she shrugged it off. 'Of course – take in any and all offers, then come back to us. That's how it works. Top offer is the best offer. Best way to look at it.'

'When you say "us",' Freya said, 'are you talking about me and my dad, or does that somehow include you?'

Levison and Solomon shared a look; the latter laughed first. 'That's my girl! All business, I told you. That's the way it's done. Look at her, isn't she gorgeous?'

'She is,' Levison agreed. 'Amazing bone structure. And those eyes... Now where have I seen those before, eh?'

Solomon looked abashed. Almost like a normal father, struggling to take a compliment, Freya thought.

'Mind you, in terms of photoshoots, you might want to consider changing the hair colour.'

'Excuse me?' Freya almost choked on a mouthful of wine.

'It's an honest opinion, one professional to another. It's OK – the blonde suits you, suits your style. Part of me would consider it for the sake of contrast, but contrast isn't what you need. Imagine you and your dad on the front of a weekend supplement, or the cover of a book. We need to draw people in. You suited black very well – I can see you both in black, in fact. Goes with the eyes.'

'And the eyebrows,' Solomon said, 'though I don't have the hair any more.'

'Yeah, we can do something about your eyebrows, too, sweetie.' Levison turned back to Freya. 'You've got something of the Italian widow about you, bit like Asia Argento. You know who she is? It's such a distinctive look. I mean when I first met you, you were more like Siouxsie Sioux, you know? And fair play. But you've got that something about you. Something dark and mysterious. Mysterious as death. You know that, right? Boys must tell you that all the time. You've been hiding it behind all these weird colours, and it's a look, I'll give you that. But you're more... what's the word?'

'Incredulous, is the word,' Freya said, dabbing at the side

of her mouth. 'Let's forget about talk of deals and contracts, please. I'm still trying to get my head around this situation. I'm not sure I ever will. So I think we can hold our horses, with all this.' She felt a surge of anger, and went with it. 'Incidentally, I'll wear what I like, when I like. God, are you actually my mother?'

Solomon laughed hard at this. Levison, again, might have been talking about the weather. 'As I say. Advice from one professional to another. Anyway. However it turns out, I think we can all do well out of this.'

'Especially when the police force settles up,' Solomon said. 'Which they will.'

'I think there's another question needs answering.' Freya looked directly at her father. 'Who's the killer?'

'That's somebody else's problem.'

'I mean, I know this will have occurred to you before now, but… They already fit you up for June Caton-Bell's murder. They've got four more they can fit you up for. And a cynic might say… There's a lot of circumstantial evidence tying you to those ones, too.'

Solomon paused. 'True. But not enough to bring charges – no forensics, no witnesses, nothing. So, it's unlikely they'll bring charges now. And it's much harder these days to fit someone up, with all the forensic science available. It's probably changed since I went inside. And – you're forgetting these new lasses. The ones who disappeared this year. Now, what everyone can agree upon is – I couldn't have done those ones.'

'So the guy who did the new murders… he's still on the loose?'

'It could be a copycat. Or it could be the real Woodcutter.

It doesn't much matter, as far as we're concerned.' He looked into her eyes. 'But I'd be worried, if I was you, frankly. You're not safe.'

'The police have been all over it,' Freya said, dismissively.

'You know, I'm staying somewhere safe,' Solomon said, in a more serious tone. There was something about the way his eyes caught the light, when the lines in his face relaxed a little, that utterly fascinated Freya. 'They're probably watching me, too, but all the same – offer's there. There's enough room, where I am. And if there's someone out there wanting to take a swing at you again, well... he'll have me to deal with.'

'Not necessary. But thank you. I'm presuming they're watching my flat. So, I'm probably safer than I've ever been. Personally, I do think the guy who contacted me is the real Woodcutter. But I don't know for sure, so we can't rule out a copycat. But there are other theories on the go. I'm sure you know them all.'

'We've got all night,' Levison said. 'Let's hear them.'

'OK.' Freya cleared her throat, and leaned forward. 'There's one theory that says not all the Woodcutter killings were carried out by the same person. That's one that intrigues me. That they might not be a series of killings after all – more like some random attacks with similarly messy consequences. A bit like they say about Jack the Ripper – there's a theory that there isn't a "canonical five" there, at all. There's another theory that June Caton-Bell was murdered to make it *look* like the Woodcutter got her. I'm sure there's other weird and wonderful ones I haven't got around to. And there'll be more to come out, once all the forensic work is complete. Hopefully that'll take us closer to the truth. Because there is an answer in there, somewhere. My God, that must be a busman's holiday at the pathology department. Four brand-new jigsaw puzzles to complete. Can you imagine?'

Solomon barked laughter. 'Hey... You might be onto something there.' He signalled a waiter. 'Champagne please. The most expensive bottle you have.'

This broke Levison's composure. 'Uh, make that the third-most expensive bottle you have, in fact. We're celebrating, but we're not millionaires. Not yet.'

'Understood, ma'am,' the waiter said, a study in discretion.

Solomon cheered when the bottle was popped – giving Freya the first 'please don't, Dad – I can't believe you' moment of her life. Her glass was filled, and the treacherous bubbles tickled her all the way down.

'Cheers!' Solomon said, as they clinked glasses again. 'To freedom. To success. And to us.'

Freya was gulping down the champagne, wondering what starter she might have out of the bewildering list of foodstuffs in front of her, when the chair next to her slid out.

Bernard Galvin's flat-nosed face peered over the top of a menu. 'Bloody starving, me. Do they do fish and chips in here, love?'

49

Cheryl Levison sprang from her seat. For a moment Freya was sure she was going to run across the table to physically tackle the newcomer.

'What are you doing here?' she yelled. 'This is a private dinner, and you aren't invited.'

'Settle down, love. As it happens, I have a booking. Just happens to be the same time as you.'

'Yeah, that'll be right – out. Now.'

Every face in the restaurant was turned towards them; every conversation stilled.

'I just want to talk. You can behave yourself, love.'

'Call me "love", one more time. Just once more.'

'C'mon, now,' Galvin said, his grey eyes passing from Levison to Solomon. 'There's no need for unpleasantness. We're all on the same side here, aren't we?'

Levison stood in between Solomon and Galvin's seats. 'You'll have to convince me of that, Bernard. Make it quick. This is a decent place. Let's not have a scene.'

'Only one causing a scene is you, Miss Levison.'

Solomon didn't move. His features became quizzical, edging towards bemused. He affected relaxation, but had his body fully turned towards Galvin. His glass was cradled between his middle fingers, and the bottle of champagne was an inch or two from his left hand. 'Stunning coincidence, you turning up, Bernie,' he said. 'And on your own, too. Haven't you got a date?'

Galvin smiled, mirthlessly. 'Looks like she skipped out on me.'

'Shame. You've got no luck with the girls.'

'I just wanted to talk. That's all. You can relax, Miss Levison.' Galvin stressed the honorific with the impudence of a child. Although she'd already seen him cave in Mick Harvie's face, this was the first moment Freya wondered if he was truly deranged or not. Her legs quivered with tension, and her bladder seemed to shrink with every passing moment. 'Sit down, please. I'm not here for a fight. Mind if I have some champagne?'

Solomon moved his hand to cover the bottle; Levison got closer to Galvin as he did so. 'I very much mind,' Levison said.

'As you please. Tad expensive in here, all the same. So, what we having, then?' Galvin raised a menu and affected nonchalance. He raised his eyebrows, turning the pages. 'Some of this is a right mouthful. I thought a roulade was something you played?'

'Just hurry up and say what you've come to say,' Levison snarled. 'This is a night of celebration. You're not celebrating, are you?'

'Could be,' Galvin said. 'I could be celebrating very soon.'

'Tomorrow morning, I'm going to apply for a restraining order against you,' Levison said. 'It'll be a very detailed proceeding, and I have to tell you – I'm going to enjoy it.'

'You're a fair lass for details. I came to congratulate you, in fact. Well done.' He extended a hand for Solomon to shake.

'That's very kind of you,' Solomon said, clearing his throat. He did not accept the handshake, but stood up, instead. He took the bottle of champagne by the neck. 'Will you join us in a toast? Grab a glass, Bernard. I'll get you some champagne. It's the third-most expensive in the house, I understand.'

Galvin smiled, and dropped his hand from the table. Freya hardly dared breathe.

'No? Shame.' Solomon placed the champagne back in the ice bucket, and got to his seat. 'You not wanting to drink my health?'

'I wish you good health,' Galvin said. 'Because I want you to stay healthy.'

'Got plans for me, have you?' Solomon grinned.

'Oh yeah. Back to jail. That's my plan for you. Finding the evidence that puts you away for good.' Galvin turned to Freya. 'This guy here – your father… I told you about him already. That time you came over with the ace newshound. I'll say it to his face. I said to him at the time. I said it when I interviewed him.'

'That's when you slapped me, wasn't it?' Solomon said. 'It's true. He did slap me. That part of the interview tape mysteriously disappeared. Not a well-known fact, but definitely a fact. Right across the face. Crack! I can still hear it even now.'

'Not nearly hard enough,' Galvin said. He laid down the menu. 'As I was saying, Freya. Your dad here – a special case. There's a lot of stuff we found out about him that didn't appear in the trial. Didn't appear on your boyfriend's daft little website, either.'

Solomon sighed. 'Bernie, if there's something you want to get off your chest…'

'Your dad went out of his way to collect snuff movies. People being killed. Young women, mostly. He even had – get this – 8mm film of a woman being raped and murdered. I sat there and watched it with my own eyes.'

'That was planted,' Solomon said. 'Along with the magazines you allegedly found. They couldn't prove that stuff was mine. I'd been in my digs for about a week, when I got arrested. So you're lying, Bernard. Like you lied about a lot of things.'

'Amazing coincidence, eh?' Galvin said. 'You had a good lawyer, I'll give you that. Got a lot of that struck out. Couldn't prove it was yours. Strange that it should all be hidden in a room let out to a serial killer, though.'

'I'd best ask my legal eagle – Cheryl, was that libel?'

'Slander,' Levison said. 'Slander is spoken, libel is written. He said it out loud. In front of a lot of people.'

'And then,' Galvin continued, 'there's the fact that he was around a lot of the sites where those people were snatched. Awfully convenient.'

'As you say – coincidence,' Solomon said. 'But while you're thinking out loud, can you talk us through the recent cases? You know anything about those?'

'Absolutely nothing,' Galvin said, amiably. 'That's someone else's problem. Someone else's murders. Fair play – I know you didn't do those ones.'

'The real Woodcutter did,' Freya said. 'The guy you

should have been looking for. The guy you should have arrested and jailed. Not my dad.'

'Oh, I know who the Woodcutter is. Fairly sure of it. It's only a matter of proof. And I think the proof's coming. I can almost feel it.' Galvin grinned at Levison. 'That all legally fair and square, Miss Levison?'

'I prefer Ms Levison.'

'Mizzzz Levison. Got you.'

'Now, try not to say it as if you had a mouthful of marbles.'

'I won't take up any more of your time,' Galvin took a breath, and placed a hand in his coat, as if he had discovered a pain somewhere in his ribs. 'I just wanted you to know I'm around, Gareth. I'm retired now, you know – got plenty of time on my hands.'

'Wife gone, too?' Solomon said.

'Dead,' Galvin said, turning his dull grey gaze on Solomon.

'Shame. It wasn't me, before you ask.'

There was a moment of silence, before Galvin laughed aloud. He slammed his hands down on the table. 'Ha! Always was a joker, this one. I'll say that for him. And a ladies' man. You watch yourself with him, Mizzz Levison. Your client's a ladykiller, you might say.'

'Oh – speaking of ladies. How's Carol Ramirez doing?' Solomon asked.

'Halfway to Timbuktu, on a very slow boat, last I heard,' Galvin said. 'Why do you ask?'

'Just wondering. You might know more than me, that's all. Getting her put away, and all. Nice work, that. Still working out whether that one was strictly legal, aren't we?' Solomon said.

Galvin turned to Freya. 'You know, dear, your dad here… he has his way with women. That's the truth. We'll never know what your mother thought of him – if she thought much of anything. But there's a really strange pattern with all his other girlfriends over the years. He has a habit of turning them absolutely doolally. Now I admit, that's not a politically correct term these days, but it's striking, all the same. I remember Carol Ramirez when she was a young PC – a WPC, I think we still called them, back then. Outstanding officer. Fearless. Then she met Solomon, and all of a sudden she's a mental case. Secure unit. Strange, isn't it? There's another lass from the late Eighties who's still scared to leave the house. Another lass from schooldays who ran away from him when he took her out into the woods one day. Another couple in a car pulled up to help when she ran into the road, screaming. Couldn't be made to talk about it. Gareth here said it was a lover's tiff.'

'We're all young once, Bernie. Even you,' Solomon said. 'You've had rows with people. That time you're talking about – that was an argument we had, when I said I couldn't see her any more. She went crazy. We had a row – but who hasn't had a row? You've had plenty of them. Carol told me that you used to enjoy shouting and screaming at people. Not averse to using your fists, either. I think they called it "old-school", till recently. Then they started calling it assault, bullying, abuse. You retired early, Bernie, is that right? Took early retirement?'

Galvin said nothing.

'Yeah,' Solomon went on, 'and I know about your eye

for outstanding PCs. Carol was outstanding, no question of that. Spanish eyes. I loved that about her. Raven-haired. She had to work at keeping the moustache under control, electrolysis and what have you. But still. What a woman. You ever see a bush like that on pale skin in the moonlight, Galvin? I know it wasn't for lack of trying. You had Carol pinned up against a wall, I'm told. Not even considering "no" for an answer. Helping yourself to handfuls. Until she kneed you right in the knackers. Plenty of backlift, too. Right down the fairway. Apparently, Bernie here was on the floor, bent double, yelping like a docked fucking spaniel.'

Solomon's eyes were huge, dark, forbidding pools.

He went on: 'I wish I could have seen that. And then... Well. Next thing you know, Carol's in a secure unit, and can't give evidence at my trial. To be fair, she was actually crazy. Death kick. Very unsavoury stuff. And then there's the arson. She scared me, truth to tell. Just as well she was institutionalised – God knows what might have happened had I dumped her and moved on. Like I was going to. But lucky me, I got arrested, so that put a capper on things.'

Galvin folded, then unfolded a napkin on the table. 'You're a filthy liar. You're as wrong as wrong can get, Gareth, and you've got no place in civilised society alongside civilised people. The world will know it before I'm finished living in it.'

'And you're a bully and a boor, who got caught fabricating evidence,' Solomon hit back. 'I don't hold out much hope for justice catching up with you, but soon the whole world will be talking about what you did, and what you didn't do. You'll be the poster boy for police corruption, if you aren't already. The guy who fabricated a case, and let a serial killer get away with it. So, think on that.'

Galvin got up. 'As you please, son. I'm all in, though. To the finish. That's all.'

'Hey – let's make a date,' Solomon said, in a lower tone of voice.

'You what?'

'I said, let's make a date. For two minutes' time. Outside. You and me.'

Levison raised a hand. 'This has gone on far enough. Bernie, get outside, or I'll call the police.'

'I believe you, Gareth,' Galvin said. 'You're serious. You must have gotten tough inside. Must be a fair old workout, trying to stay healthy with the lifers. Lots of unbelievably bad things can happen to a guy like you in prison.'

'Worse things happen to bent coppers,' Solomon said.

Galvin unbuttoned his coat and reached inside.

Solomon was out of his seat, fast; Freya barely saw him lift the champagne bottle.

Levison was swifter than both of them. Before Freya could see her move, she had seized Galvin by the lapels, dragging his grey anorak-style coat off his shoulders and restricting the movement of his arms.

Then Galvin's face dripped red.

Freya had flipped her original wine glass. It still had a fair volume of red in it. All of which went over Galvin's face.

There were cries of alarm and consternation. Two waiters appeared, then a manager in a suit. Galvin was bustled out, trying to twist himself free of the waiters. His grey anorak was stained through with fresh blossoms of wine, some big, some small.

As the unwieldy quartet bustled out of the huge double doors into the stark white corridor, there was an ugly, telltale sound of a fist hitting flesh.

Solomon was doubled over, laughing. Levison was still on her feet, parsing the situation, taking in all the shocked faces. 'It's fine,' she said, to no one in particular. 'Totally fine. Everything's fine.'

'Great shot,' Solomon said at last, raising a thumb in Freya's direction. 'Bang on the button. That's vengeance, right there. That's my girl!'

Freya got up, and waved at an ashen-faced waitress at the bar. 'Hey,' she said, as the girl reluctantly came to join her, 'is there a back door out of here?'

'Not staying?' Solomon asked.

'Sorry, Dad. Lost my appetite a bit.'

Before she left, she picked up something that had landed on the table, almost unnoticed. It was the thing Galvin had been reaching into his pocket for; it had fluttered out of his grasp like a moth circling a bulb, and landed on the table before Freya. She pocketed it as she got up. It was Galvin's card.

50

'Where are you going?'

Levison chased her through the metal guts of the restaurant, the secret chambers where food bathed under hot lights, fat sizzled, and wraiths in white yelled at each other.

Freya kept walking, until she was shown to a fire escape. She finally turned to face Levison when she was outside, in an anti-courtyard filled with pipes, fire escapes, wheelie bins and one overflowing skip. It was as if a respectable building had been turned inside out, perhaps at gunpoint, with all its dirty corners exposed.

'Hey! Freya!'

Freya turned to face her. 'Thanks for a pleasant evening, Cheryl,' she said, brightly.

Levison stood out like a dove on a tarred roof with her white dress – still irritatingly pristine, despite red wine having been erupted mere inches away. 'Don't get cute. Why are you running away? Do you know what you were offered, in there?'

Freya folded her arms. 'The keys to your kingdom. Not mine.'

'You think you can do better?' Levison grew haughty.

'Listen. You're clever. But you're young. You don't know it all. You've been offered a deal in there, and I would strongly advise you to take it.'

'I haven't refused anything,' Freya spluttered. 'You've just run after me here in your high heels, after subjecting me to some of the worst unarmed combat I've ever seen between two middle-aged men – and let me tell you, that's a pretty high bar. Now you're sneering at me for not accepting some non-existent offer. Why don't you speak the truth, Cheryl? You didn't come out here to chivvy me about a book deal. I'll take your book deal. We can even shake on it now, if you like. But that's not what you want to tell me. So, spit it out.'

Levison faltered, and folded her arms. It was as close as she came to being discomfited, or anything less than an Olympian-grade hard case. 'I had hoped we could do it in private, some other time. But you're right. It's fair enough that I tell you. Withholding it isn't fair.'

'I'm listening.'

'I can't say to you, in all confidence, that your father isn't a serial killer.'

Freya wanted to laugh. 'That's it? That's your big secret? That there's a slight doubt about the guy?'

'I thought it was only fair to tell you.'

'Is this something you think, or something you know?'

'I can't breach client confidentiality.'

'He's told you that he did it? He admitted it to you?'

Levison shook her head. 'I shouldn't have said anything. No, for the record, he didn't do that. I've said all I wanted to say. I couldn't let you go without telling you.'

Freya shrugged. 'This hasn't changed anything. For what

it's worth, I believe he's innocent. Maybe I'm projecting goodness that isn't there? Who knows?'

'I'm sorry, Freya. For what it's worth… I don't think this affects how we continue with this project in any way. And I haven't told Gareth. I was considering not telling you at all, but that's unethical. I think you've been through some horrible things in a very short space of time, and there's no telling what psychological damage it could do to you if you found out something new about Gareth. But you deserve to know. He's not right.'

'Unethical, you say. But we're still going ahead with books and interviews and probably TV and radio appearances. Would that be right?'

'We've still to discuss all that.'

'That's a lawyer's answer, all right.'

'It's all I can tell you for now. I'm sorry, Freya. You look absolutely done in. I'm sorry I sprang it on you like this. It was maybe a mistake. I'll take you home. Gareth and I can drop you off.'

'No thanks.'

'Freya.' She came forward and placed both hands on the younger woman's shoulders. 'I know this isn't a comfort to you. Your mother's death, I'm not sure you've totally dealt…'

'Don't dare mention her. Don't you dare!' Freya tore herself free, then – she could never explain why, later – on impulse, she spat at Levison. 'Get that tested!'

She strode away, finding the right alleyway, where she'd left her bike chained up.

51

Her head felt as if it was floating several yards above the rest of her body as she flew through the streets on her bike. Shops, lit windows, and the usual kaleidoscope of night visions seemed especially forbidding the cosier they looked. One couple kissing, slowly, in the window of a kebab shop; three portly old men, all frozen open-mouthed at the same punchline at a pub; a woman and two girls sat on a sofa in a front room, entranced by the soft blue curtain of the television.

Freya laughed aloud at the ludicrous situation. Possibly she had misjudged Cheryl Levison, after all. She'd looked so sincere, too. Right up until the moment she spat on her. *And what's next? What new things will there be to discover? What's the end of all this?*

A car blared its horn at her as she cut across a junction, just a little bit too late for the signal opposite changing to red. She thrilled to the lights as they slashed across her pistoning legs, the faces twisted in fury on the dashboards as she forced them to brake. She carried on, at one point on the wrong side of the road, delighted by the oncoming headlights and the shriek of horns. One quick leap and she was on the pavement, going faster. It occurred to her to tear off her helmet and use it as a grenade, gaining enough spin and propulsion to force it through a pane of glass.

One teenager actually took a swing at her as she went past, but missed by a long way – and then she reached the green gates of the park.

Someone had lit a fire somewhere inside the park, and dark bodies rose to see her as she pedalled through the broad, pleasant walkways. Freya wondered what sort of figure she must have presented, a flashing light at the front, and her lines suggested only by livid streaks of pink and yellow down the sides of her hi-vis jacket, which she had kept rolled in her bag.

'We need to think about this, don't we?' she said to herself. 'We need to think about this very carefully indeed.'

Freya took a turn down past a section where there were no streetlights. The lane where she usually began her run. She might have found this stretch if she had been blindfolded – it wasn't a well-travelled path, and was overgrown at the best of times. Tonight the foliage seemed to spring back at her approach. At the top of the lane was a turnstile that gave onto more houses and led the way to her flat at the top of the road.

She eased down on the speed, allowing her headlamp to light the uneven path. Whenever it rained this path could be treacherous, sucking hard on the tyres and providing no end of laundry if she ran – but tonight, after dark, it was dry and dusty.

Her headlight picked out something shiny on the ground. Freya disregarded it; then there was another one. She slowed down a little, and saw that there was a trail of shiny things, all the way up the path. Coins, she saw; one- and two-pound coins.

'Hallo,' she said, slowing down. There seemed to be cash strewn across the path, and right up the verge. Here and there was some silver; then, caught in some grass, there were some brown and blue notes. A fair amount of them, it appeared.

Freya braked to a stop. She hesitated, checking there was no one following in front or behind, and no one looming among the trees. She felt exposed for a moment, her speed sacrificed. But someone had dropped a lot of money here.

Her first instinct was suspicion.

Then she saw the purse lying just a few yards away. A golden clasp against dark brown leather.

An accident? Someone had dropped it in a hurry.

Maybe an assault?

She might see a body peeking out from between the bushes a little further up. But there was no sign of any feet protruding from any foliage, no arms wrapped around the trees that fringed the pathway. Freya gripped the purse, stooping somewhat to do so. There'd be a name in there – she could turn it into the police tomorrow, plus all the money.

No sooner had her hand closed around the leather than something bit her, hard, around the calf muscle of her right leg. For one absurd moment she thought: *shark!*

It enclosed her whole leg; then there was a smart snapping sound, and then the world spun about. Everything was inverted; the black of the night traded positions with the forest; blood surged to her head.

The bike fell, the back wheel spinning, and the light

splashing across the brown dirt path. She was off the ground, and upside down.

Whatever had bit her, bit down harder. She flailed and thrashed, then reached up towards the source of the pain.

It was a rope. She had been snared.

'Oh no,' was all she could say, 'oh no, oh no, oh no, you must be joking…'

'No joke,' said a grating voice.

She heard him, but didn't see him, until he was right upon her. She swiped and clawed at the sudden, terrifying shadow, so dense as to swallow even night, but there was no impact. Freya swung in the air like a pendulum.

Something snapped over her face; her breath was caught within it, and the world misted over. A face mask. She screamed, but it was totally muffled, and two hands caught hold of her hands, tight, stopping the swaying.

'That's it,' someone said. 'We're nearly home, now. Almost there.'

The voice faded. Freya couldn't even have sworn that she was entirely unconscious, but the night, the spinning wheel, the headlight and the bright green grasses it illuminated faded away.

52

Hello there! Well. This is a treat, and no mistake. No mistake!

Whoa. Drove a little bit too fast, there. Don't want to get stopped by the cops. Not tonight, of all nights! Whew. I'm excited. Probably I should calm down. Let's all take it easy, eh?

Your head will feel a bit fuzzy. Things will seem strange. Sights, sounds… Take a moment, as they say these days. Come around. Get some deep breaths.

And don't struggle, or I will split you lengthwise.

You know, I've never done that before to someone? Not longitudinally. Transversely, yes. Half and half, yes. What a job that was! The two bodies in the weir, I did it to both of them. You ever see that film, The Pit And The Pendulum*? Oh, they saw it coming, too. They both got it. Lovely job, both of them. My peak. Until tonight, maybe? I love my work. Absolutely love my work.*

And whatever you do, don't scream. It hurts my ears, and there's just no need. OK?

Don't struggle, I said. Don't bang the side of the van. It'll be disappointing to stop and just cut your throat, but that's what I'll do if you give me any trouble.

Either of you.

Just sit there quietly, take some deep breaths, and conserve energy. All right? That's the best thing for you to do. Keep something in reserve. You're going to need it.

You are in a very privileged position. Not many folk in your shoes actually get to live the dream, you know? It's exciting for me, too. I was reading that website of yours, Freya. You and the gormless-looking bastard with the glasses. You know the guy I mean. You've been so, so busy. You did so well with the clues. But you must've known this night would come. Surely you got yourself ready for it? Mentally, at least. You must have known I'd come for you. Took a lot of studying. Checking your route. You take a risk going through that path, day or night, let me tell you. Some nerve. You might meet some right evil bastard one night! Hah!

And as for you, *my lovely… You get to be in on it. Further than you ever thought possible. I wonder if you thought Solomon was the one, after all? Wonder if he told you that he was?*

We've not got long to go. You've both been out for quite some time. Best that way. I do worry that something's going to go wrong, and I'm going to lose one of my people, one day.

You've been let into a secret, in fact. My MO for capturing people. They never quite figured it out. But now you both know. Yeah, that's how I did it. Same way I got you. The snare, the gas. So effective. Dodgy, but I've never lost anyone yet. Apart from the bitch I had to cosh. Screamed a bit too loudly. Had to think better of it. But by and large, it works. You're never fully unconscious, you know. Just sedated.

It's better than pulling people over, better than asking for directions, all of these things.

I stalk victims, for ages. The books and websites were right about that. I took my time, and studied routes. Like I studied yours. It's so much easier to trace someone when they travel by bike. Or if they've got a running route. If you'd taken a bus or walked the streets, it would be so much harder to get you in the back of the van. But you like going to quiet places, Freya. And that was your mistake.

So, yeah, I set the snare, then leave a trail of breadcrumbs. Banknotes, hard cash... it would make anyone *a mark. You see a tenner on the ground somewhere, you pick it up. Anyone would. Hey, I would... and I'm the fucking Woodcutter!*

Then I get busy with the gas. A nice tank of it attached to a mask. It's the same stuff you used to get at the dentist's. I make it myself these days. You don't get it so much any more, there's been a bit of a change in the law. But the good stuff, that puts you out of reach. Nice and calm, nice and quick. Too much and you can flatline, but that would be bad news for everybody. That's it, that's the trick. Snare 'em, get the mask on 'em, they're out. Bob's your auntie. That's what happened to them, that's what happened to you.

Had to be a bit more of an opportunist with you, my love. You're a smarter cookie than you look. Took more than a little chance, creeping up behind you. That's the thing about smoking, it's an underground habit, these days. Have to go into alleyways and creepy little corners to do it. Hey, you know, those things'll kill you! Ha!

Do you know, Freya, when I saw your dad in the papers, it coaxed me out of retirement? I guess you could say the new ones are your fault. When you find something you like, it's hard to give it up, eh?

And now, finally, it's your turn. Beautiful, you must admit. All ties together.

I can't wait for your specky boyfriend to find you. That's going to be a good one. I might hang around to watch that happen. I might even let him know I'm there. I like to give folks a scare. A scare you won't believe, in fact. Won't be long now!

You can't see it, but it's so dark out here. A nice moonlit night. You'll just about be able to see where you're going. And that is very important. Have you pissed yourself there, Freya? No? Smells a bit like it. That can happen, of course. Don't think it was your lawyer friend, there. It'd have shown on her dress a bit more. Ah, never mind. This piece of shit van's getting torched not long after I dump your bits and pieces. You'll leave no trace. Nothing that I don't want people to find, anyway.

We're just about here. I'll take a quick drive around, make sure there's absolutely no one here. Dog walkers pop up in all sorts of weird places. So do doggers. No joke, I had to do a U-turn once – there were all sorts of shenanigans going on in the site I'd picked. The beauty of that was, no one was going to admit to seeing a van out there, were they? Dirty bastards.

Anyway. There we are. Quick turn around… Nope, all clear. Another turn… all clear, looking good. Yep. We're clear. All alone!

Now I'll let you into another trade secret. This is how it's done. Your boyfriend's theory is correct. What I like is the chase. I let them go, then I go after them. No one's escaped, so far. Not one. But it's a fair chase. I'm going to come around and open the van door, now. You might be tempted to escape, but... you see this? Know what this is? That's right. It's a shotgun. I'm going to crack the stock, now... See that in there? That's right. Two shells. I'll put the first one in your knee, if either of you give me any trouble. Then you'll have to crawl away, rather than run. Not that it'll change the result. But it'll be less interesting for me.

Now this is the interesting part. This is where I break new ground. You're in a race for your life – with me. But you're also in a race with each other. Settle down, girls. I'll explain.

Well. Here we are. And here I am. Sorry about the mask. For the best. Just in case you get away. On the off chance.

What's that? My goodness, Freya. That language! Your father would be ashamed if he could hear you.

Please don't spit, either. Here's Mr Shotgun again. It's pointed right at the point of your knee. It'll probably take the lower leg off. Don't doubt me. All right? No more.

Good. Now. You can see where we are. This is a former quarry. There was a pit, just up over the brow of the hill, too. You might even recognise it. See that contraption up there? Looks like a dinosaur's neck? That's the former pit elevator. That's your end goal. Reach that, you're safe. Now, I can catch both of you, or just one of you. Whoever I get first, is obviously going to slow me down a little. So play this game tactically. Gads, I've been so excited about this! And here we are!

Funny old place, this. All kinds of corridors and walkways... I think they wanted this to be a nuclear site at one point. Cooling rods and what have you. They were going to expand it all, then either the money ran out or the government got a better offer. I can't remember. Anyway, here we are. Some night, eh? A good night to die. I thought I was overstretching myself, taking two on at the same time. Digging out those old bodies and planting them in the weir gave me ideas, though. You've got to test yourself, haven't you? You've got to go to the edge.

Now you have a trail around the old place – slag heaps and such. They're thinking of turning it into a nature reserve, can you believe. 'Cos they can't build houses on this land. It'll fall into hell. There are a few bunkers they built here and there, sunk into the hills. Old crates and cabins. I think even the tramps are too smart to stay in them, now.

There are many ways you can go. Trails, dips, trenches, even one or two sharp drops. It's up to you whether you pick the right way or not. Down the decline? There are pits down here, filled with water, algae, bacteria, you name it. There are coal bings and bunkers of varying types. However you choose to cross the ground towards the pit elevator is up to you. I'll be following behind. Not with the shotgun, but with this.

And finally, look what I've got here… This is it. The original and best. I've used a few, but this is the first. I kept it, especially. The one best suited to the job, too.

I sharpened it – for you especially, Freya. It's going to cut well. I think I might spare you the suffering, seeing as you've been such a good girl. I'll try to get right through your neck, first go. Or maybe between the shoulder blades – that'd do it just as quickly.

But as for you, my legal eagle… all bets are off. Understood?

The rules are – one or both of you gets to the old pit shaft elevator, you win. You stay alive. I'll leave the scene, and we'll say no more about it. I can't promise you'll find anywhere nice to sleep, and to be honest, I don't envy you a long walk through the forest in the middle of the night. Who knows where I might be hiding!

Heh. But no, seriously, you'll be free. Of course, if I catch you, then... goodnight and God bless.

Pretty simple, eh?

Any tactics you might want to employ on your fellow captive at this stage... totally up to you, girls.

I'll give you a minute to get your bearings. Once I cut the ties around your feet and hands, that's the start. You get a thirty-second head start. Make it count.

53

It was hard to speak. Freya felt as if she had been gagged, and for all she knew, she had been. Her head throbbed and her throat was sore, and when she moved her head, she felt an appalling dizziness.

Opposite her, a white and gold blur that must have been Cheryl Levison struggled against her bonds.

Freya fought nausea down, licked her lips, and tried to make out the figure before her.

He was stood in the open doorway of the van, dressed in black, his face covered by a black beanie hat. It was difficult to make out what colour his eyes were. Wherever they were, they were under an open sky, with a mechanoid monster etched against the sky over his shoulder, as much as thirty feet high. She had no idea where she was, or how long she'd been out.

Freya was laid on her back, with cable ties at her ankles, her wrists bound behind her. On top of this situation, there was the crude threat of the shotgun barrels, pointed straight at her. In his other hand was a long-handled fire axe, with a red blade and a silver-sharp shiny edge. He could have blown her in half at the twitch of a finger. If he was more at his leisure, he could have chopped off a foot with a single swipe. She didn't doubt he was capable.

The voice was more of a puzzle. Was it possible to have a portable voice changer fixed to a mask? It had to be so, though she couldn't envisage how it worked in any practical sense. It made the voice porcine and grotesque, out here in the open. Freya was reminded of a previous partner who'd snored appallingly, so much so that she had opted to sleep on the couch, and then never went back, on account of it.

'Guessed who I am yet?'

She shook her head. With full consciousness, now she felt the fear. Her heartbeat was out of control; even in the gloom she could now make out the veins ridged across the back of her hands. She doubted she could run. Apart from a stream of curses, she doubted she could speak.

'I don't believe that, you know,' he said. 'You're a clever cookie. Haven't you heard anything from our friends in the police? Some of those sources you've got? There's a lot of doubt that it's the same killer. Well, there's no doubt, I can tell you.'

'I don't believe you.' She had meant to sound defiant, but it was a squeak, a series of dry clicks. Could she be brave ever again? Could anyone. 'Show me your face. I'll tell you if I was right.'

The pig-voice laughed.

'You're not Solomon,' Levison said. She was openly biting at the cable ties across her wrists, to no avail. Her eye make-up was streaming across her face, but there was something ferocious about this smudged aspect and even wilder hair – something of the warrior. 'I know that for a fact.'

'You can't be sure though, can you? Height, body shape… voice is not giveaway…' He chuckled again.

'You could be Bernie Galvin,' Freya croaked.

The amplified laughter hurt her ears. 'It wasn't him! I can guarantee you that,' the masked figure croaked. 'So, guess again. The original idea was to give your dear old dad a few months' grace to find his feet, then chop someone to pieces. But things got the better of me. Things moved too fast. So I've gone for the star prize. You should be proud. In a way.'

'Then I give up.' Freya was out of options. Guile was not going to work. *I'm going to have to run for my life. And what're the odds of him telling the truth?*

Or I can fight. I'll find something to fight with.

Was that possible? Could she really do that? Out here, in the dark, with this nightmare?

But he is going to make me run. And Freya could run. That meant a chance. But she could not run blindly. She would assess where she was, and take a chance. If she had to face him, she'd make it awkward.

He'll shoot me. There's no way he'd have let the former squaddie get a head start on him without some unfair advantage. No way he could have made him run in the first place, without a gun.

Fine. He'll shoot me. He'll have to make me stand still first.

She tried to hold on to this feeling, gritting her teeth against it. Her wiring quivered along the muscles of her arms, back and shoulders. She felt the potential energy building in every sinew; and then, as soon as this thought cleared her mind, her calf muscles cramped, and she cried out.

A low bass chuckle. 'Point your toes up. That'll do it. Sorry. That isn't an advantage I wanted for myself, there. I had to tie you up. Hope you understand.'

'Fuck you,' Freya wheezed. But she did as he said, and the lightning bolt of pain up her leg muscle relented. She blinked, tried to focus again.

'Now, here's the thing. I'm going to cut your ties. Don't forget I have the shotgun. I'll back off. You try to run past me, to the top of the hill, and I'll bring you down. One or both of you. You can doubt this all you want, and try it if you like. But that's what'll happen. Game over. And then you're in pieces. You've got one direction to take. Run down the hill, towards the quarry, and then you're in business. For a little while, anyway. I'm faster than I look.

'Here it comes, now. I'm cutting your leg ties. Freya first. If you're tempted to kick me in the balls, don't. Look at the shotgun barrels. That's it. Good. Now your hands. There you go. Take a stretch, I don't mind. Get the circulation going. It all helps. You should see it, when the blood jets out. Nothing like it. Hey, you're all limbered up already. Excellent. Now you, counsellor. Oh, don't look at me like that. Be like Freya. Look at the shotgun. Look at where my finger is. That's it. I honestly thought you'd do it, counsellor. I thought you'd do it. Now. Both out the van. Slowly. With your hands up. That's good. In your own time, then. You ready?'

54

Freya slid her feet onto the ground. She was in a transit van of some kind – ancient, battle-scarred, possibly from an actual battlefield. Cheryl Levison pulled herself out. They both stood outside, their hands raised, breath steaming up in the cool air.

The Woodcutter gave them plenty of room. 'Your time has started,' he said. 'I'd get moving, if I was you.'

Freya did.

She ran around to the front, and tugged on the driver's side door of the van.

Locked.

He laughed. 'Nice one! This is going to be interesting. Good try. No luck, though.'

'Get moving!' Levison said. 'Head for the dips – there's more of a path there. Straight up the middle is too steep!' Then she tore off, long legs slashing her white skirt.

Freya took a breath, taking in the view before her. The site the Woodcutter had taken them to was a bowl in the earth, made of what seemed to be crumbling earth and shingle. Concentric curves wound their way through the hillside towards a central point, where there was a suggestion of the crane he had mentioned.

Freya ran, taking the right-hand path, rather than plunging down into the centre of the quarry. Stones dislodged under her feet, and she stumbled, alarmingly, crying out.

Levison was already out of sight.

How long had passed? Ten seconds? Fifteen?

She continued skirting the edge of the quarry. The lip of the quarry wound round soon enough; she could make out the detail of the gigantic industrial lifting machine, the logo and livery that remained on the side, the patches of rust on the plating. Easy, she thought. Too easy.

Almost as soon as the thought had cleared her mind, she saw the defile in the ground that had been entirely hidden by the waves of loose stone – more of a fissure, a collapsed part of the ground, cracked a long way to the right, tumbling down towards the slick black water at the bottom of the quarry. The gap was tantalising, but there was no way she could jump it; the sides were steep, and filled with loose stones, some of them broad and shiny as a new shovel.

'Bastard,' Freya hissed, and turned, and started down the side of the quarry. That was his intention, surely; to force her to take the longer, more treacherous route, down the hill.

Was Levison lying? To make sure I was behind her?

Freya used the betrayal, biting down hard, loose stones and scree rustled under her feet, and she slithered down it twice, skinning the palm of her hand, before regaining her footing. She glanced over her shoulder; the van was stark white against the dark, rocky hill, but there was no sign of the masked man.

Freya kept going until she reached the point where she could safely leap over the other side of the defile and reach the top. It had been a trick of perspective, a con of the light in a place of overlapping darkness, which had hidden the defile at first. Then another thought struck her: *I'm going exactly where he wants me to go. I have to change that.*

She kept going towards the bottom. Water splashed up, covering her feet and soaking the bottom of her trousers. Still no sign of him.

'This is it!' a voice hissed, shockingly close. 'This is what we wanted!'

He was right there.

He'd come down the other side of the pit. A snail-like silvery trail marked a steep, but defined path. No defile there. A flash of metal, constrained movement released, then the whistling metallic arc in the air.

He was aiming for her head, and close enough to reach her.

She ran into the space where the blow was about to fall, not away, ducking low; the axe blade whirled over her head.

Freya followed through, and butted him somewhere in the midriff. He crashed to the ground. She looked for the axe; not fast enough; flare of silver as he snatched up again, scrambling to his feet, then he swung it again, aiming for her ankle. He just missed.

She ran on impulse, straight up the hill, where the head of the pit elevator bent towards her. Benevolent. A plant-eating dinosaur. She scrambled up the stones – no two ways about it, Levison had surely made the checkpoint. It was just her and him, and she had a chance, unless he had one more problem in store for her, one more shock...

Freya reached the top of the hill, the backs of her thighs aching, but all her training was paying off. She was not aware of fatigue, just a heightened state of awareness born of adrenaline. She did not even look back as she sprinted towards the lip of the quarry, with the gleaming promise of the pit lift up ahead. All she had to do was reach it – or so he said.

Freya had maybe forty yards to cover. She couldn't hear any footsteps behind her.

That's when her leading foot landed on nothing; she was falling into space, momentum carrying her through another gap in the earth. Her hands clasped on nothing; the gap was a good ten feet, utterly invisible until she was right on it.

Freya curled into a ball; she rebounded off the cleft in the quarry, stones and earth streaming off her shoulder and trickling against her face. She collided with loose stones, taking most of the impact on her wrists and shin. No way to tell up or down, left or right, and she fell for a time before the natural slope of the cut in the quarry arrested her fall.

Freya stopped rolling at the bottom of the slope, cut, winded, shocked. The throbbing at her fingertips and at her knuckles and elbows foretold incredible pain to come, but she wasn't bleeding too badly and she could still move.

She did; she clawed her way back up a near-vertical slope. When a flickering light appeared just above her, she screamed.

This was it. He had somehow outflanked her, even as she fell down this fresh pit. Of course he had. He'd wanted her to come this way. Freya had followed his design perfectly. He had studied his killing ground well. There was no choice. There had been no option for lateral thinking, no dodge, no emergency exit.

The light she glimpsed was surely from a candle, burning in a box cut into the earth. It looked like a bunker of some kind, with a rectangular window denuded of glass. It resembled nothing less than an old coach or train carriage, set into the earth – some kind of canteen or clubhouse or even office. It looked like it had moved, or been partly buried, thanks to subsidence.

Rocks crumbled somewhere above. She perceived movement without actually seeing it, in the extreme left of her visual field.

If he knew about this pit, and he surely did, he would have outflanked her on the left-hand side, and was probably waiting for her at the top.

The flickering yellow light in the bunker surely meant death for Freya, but her choices were limited. She climbed towards it.

The bunker hung over a fresh dip, somewhat precariously balanced. As she got closer, she saw that it was corrugated, like a shipping container, and badly rusted. She tensed, gripped the edges of the empty window frame. There was no glass remaining to slice her fingertips. Freya took the strain on her shoulders, her feet perched on the edge of the defile, and pulled herself inside.

She landed inside the bunker – not as quietly as she would have liked. The floor was covered in earth. That aside, the candle burned on a wooden table, beside a set of wooden packing crates and, bizarrely, a brass bedstead covered with a filthy mattress. Whatever once covered the walls had long been reclaimed by earth and mould.

Freya pulled out the wooden crates, but there was

something inside them and she struggled to move them, her lower back aching. She gave up, and turned to the bed.

'Fuck it,' she hissed, and dropped and rolled underneath it.

She heard stones crumble outside, and for a moment she entertained a horrible notion that the entire structure was going to tip out into the quarry, dislodged by Freya's movement inside.

Freya gripped ancient metal spokes underneath the bed frame, and pulled herself off the ground. Turning her head, she had a full view of the empty window.

A lithe figure raised itself over the lip of the portal, and grunted as it raised itself inside. It dropped onto its haunches with barely any sign of discomfort, got to its feet, and walked into the light.

Cheryl Levison.

55

Levison's dress was in shreds, and Freya noticed that her feet were bare, smeared with soot, grime and blood. Levison's eyes showed no surprise. She crossed over to the flickering candle, and immediately snuffed it out. Only a cool moonlight remained, casting a thin, shiny blade across the floor.

Then she limped over to the bed. Freya shrunk back, still trying to process what she was seeing from the bottom. It seemed impossible that Levison hadn't seen her hiding under there.

Freya let her back touch the floor again.

Levison gripped the bed. Freya did not know whether to speak, or to cover her mouth and nose to muffle her heavy breathing.

The bed shifted. Then, barely audible: 'Freya, if you're there…'

'Cheryl,' Freya croaked.

Levison still leapt in fright. 'Thank God. I thought you were in here. Listen – we've got every chance if we pair up. We can both take him down, and finish it tonight. I'll see if one of these boxes…'

Freya edged out from underneath the bed on her elbows.

Levison had moved towards the packing crates, attempting to move them aside. 'These are heavy,' she grunted. 'There might be something we can use for a weapon.'

'The top one's empty,' Freya said. 'We can break it up, use the wood as a club.'

'That's as good an idea as any,' Levison said. She blew a stray lock of hair away from her forehead, and smiled. Freya felt a burst of confidence. He couldn't tackle two of them.

They both heard it clearly. The sound of a lock turning. A door grated open behind the packing crates.

'Boo!' said a familiar voice.

Freya shrank back under the bed.

There was the sound of a dull, heavy connection. Levison sprawled back on the floor. Blood gushed from a wound on her chest, dark and glistening in the thin light. Levison was turned to face Freya, mouth open.

Then two gloved hands gripped her by the lapels. Levison was hurled on top of the bed with tremendous force. The bedstead crashed back against the wall, the springs bounded off Freya's face, and she compressed herself back against the wall, as far as she could. All she could see were Cheryl Levison's bare feet dangling off the end of the bed, and two booted feet stomping towards her.

She quite clearly saw the axe head, held low, stained along the edge where it had crashed into Levison's chest.

'Ah I'm glad it was you, first. So glad. Been a long time coming.'

Levison gurgled, rather than screamed.

The blade disappeared. Freya saw his stance shift, his feet braced. Freya covered her mouth with her hands. Then the bed, and the wall behind it, quivered as the blade struck home.

'There! There we are!' The voice distorter had shifted to a near diabolical pitch, the sound of saw blades clashing, or an unbearable level of electronic interference.

One of Levison's feet flailed on the edge of the bed. Then he surged forward again, and the same foot was on the floor, along with half of her shin.

Freya saw the dainty ankle, the manicured toes, the red lipstick, and the floor behind spattered with blood.

'Bitch, the state of you, sneering at the world, sneering at me,' the Woodcutter raved.

Levison gurgled again, the bed thrashing, as the blade swung down again.

'Gonna *own* you!'

Then her screaming abruptly stopped.

'That's right. That's right. That's the end of it, the end,' he shrieked. The blade crashed down again, again, and again. Blood dripped through the blankets and the slats above; it pattered onto Freya's forehead, dribbling into her eyes. She shrank back further. But there was nowhere else to go.

Above, he bellowed like an animal, crashing down the axe again, and again. One brass slat split in two, its jagged edge dangling just above Freya's face. Freya saw the axe blade crash through another slat right above her head, almost passing completely through. The edge wiggled, as if in excitement or merriment, as he tugged the blade out.

Even more enraged, he chopped, chopped, and chopped. Blood pooled on the floor. She heard its insistent dripping. Then he rested the blade on the floor. It was stained right up to the top of the handle in gore.

'Now,' he wheezed. 'Now. That's that. That's one bitch down. First of a double bill. And now, folks. The main event. What you've been waiting for.'

He got to his knees. The masked face was utterly unreadable, but there was still a note of glee in his voice.

'Surprise!'

Cheryl Levison's face appeared beside his. Her blonde hair had come free during the attack, and covered most of her face, glued to the ultra-white skin by her blood. Her head had also come free during the attack, blood still oozing from the terrible wound. Only one eye showed through the strands of hair, wide open in shock and horror.

Then the head rolled across the floor as he cast it aside. And reached for Freya.

56

Freya jabbed the jagged brass slat right into his face.

She had no idea if she'd hit him in the eye, as she'd hoped, but the effect was perfect. He cried out, clutching his face, getting up to his knees. He turned to her and reached out again, but by that point she had hurtled out from beneath the bed and sprinted towards the open window space. There was a scratch at her leg from his gloves; her feet slithered in a blood smear, and she almost overbalanced. But she reached the window and clambered out.

As she edged through the narrow space, she saw him get to his feet, and snatch up the axe from the blood-slicked human disaster zone on what remained of the bed. He actually snarled as he ran forward, with the blade poised high above his head.

The blade cracked through the plaster on the sill, less than two inches from the edge of Freya's nose, biting deep into the masonry beneath.

Then she was free, tumbling onto the slope beneath.

Freya waited, her ear cocked towards the window.

She heard the sound of the packing crates shifting across the floor, then the hidden door grating open.

Freya climbed back onto the sill of the window, her toes

right on the very edge, then gripped the roof of the structure. She pulled herself on top, shoulder muscles stretched taut, and then she waited again. She heard footsteps; the structure must be connected to others inside the earth. Perhaps it was part of an old control tower, still to be demolished; a common room, or similar, facing out into the upper world. It had the look of a temporary structure, a forerunner of the kind of cabins you saw on building sites. Perhaps it had been temporarily buried when the site was decommissioned.

The surface of the bunker creaked, and gave slightly under her feet. She peered down for a second, and pushed down, cautiously. The roof was firmer, now.

Freya gazed up towards the head of the lift apparatus. It seemed to nod at her in the moonlight. That was the target; though she had no doubt that there was a surprise in store for her if she got there. She had crossed beyond the point of fear and was working on sheer adrenaline, lightning-quick connections, every nerve on edge.

She waited, to see where he would emerge. She stepped forward, heading to the far side of the roof. At one point, it creaked beneath her feet. She ground her teeth and waited, staring at what she was stepping on.

Silence followed. Then a breath of wind circulated the loose stones of the pit. It cooled the sweat on Freya's brow. She looked around for a weapon, anything to use; her hands delved into the loose stones nearby.

Then a dark shape leapt down from the angled folds in the ground above. He was at the other side of the bunker, the part that was sunk into the earth. There was the length of the roof between him and Freya. The hidden door must have opened out on the other side of the hill.

The surface of the quarry edged down sharply at the edge of the structure Freya was on, far too steep to run down. She should have stayed at the other side, and taken a circular route around the depression.

While he gibbered, Freya weighed up the stones. None of them were big enough to do much damage. She saw herself casting them at him, and having them merely bounce off.

He took a step closer. 'You have options. You can jump down that gap. You might not turn your ankle. Then again, you might. If you do, all you can do is wait until I reach you. Or you could fight. It's up to you. You have a chance.'

Freya let the stones fall to the ground. 'Bastard,' was all she could say, more of a sob than an imprecation. 'You bastard. Leave me alone.'

'Excellent! Fight it is, then!' He darted forward onto the roof of the bunker. 'Just what I always wanted!'

Then the bunker creaked. The roof gave way. And he fell.

He let the axe go on reflex, and it disappeared. Somehow, he held on, clinging to the edges of the hole that had opened up with his fingertips. But he was losing his fight with gravity. The dark, masked face bobbed into view, right at her feet. She heard him grunt with the effort of it.

Freya gawped. Just for a second.

The part of the bunker she'd stepped across… it was rusted right through. He'd gone right through the roof.

The face quivered, the gasps perhaps even more pathetic through the voice changer, as he lost his battle to hold on.

'Fight, was it?' Freya said, thickly. 'A fight, you said? Don't you move. Stay right there…'

She aimed a kick at his face; before it could connect, he

let go, and dropped into space. She heard him cry out as he hit the floor below, the room they had just left.

Freya sagged to her knees for a second, relief, horror and exhaustion hitting her simultaneously.

She gazed at the yawning hole he'd fallen through, the rusted edging where the panel had simply dropped away.

'Hope you haven't turned your ankle down there,' she said. Then she turned towards the slope above.

Above the bunker, Freya had a near-vertical part to climb, maybe four or five feet high. There were plenty of footholds in solid rock, and she clambered over it. Then the slope eased off into loose stones. It was treacherous; she was soon at the top, on flat ground. Ahead was the lift apparatus, its steel cords still reaching into the earth. The ground was overgrown, full of weeds and bushes; she ignored these as they whipped and tore at her skin. Soon she reached a covered ladder. With a dreadful jolt that drew a cry from her throat, she saw that it was covered with a hatch, with a padlock hanging from it.

She tugged the padlock. It had rusted through; the two parts separated and the padlock clinked to the concrete.

'Oh thank God! Thank you, God!'

In full panic mode now, Freya pulled open the hatch and started up the ladder. The entire structure vibrated; she had a terrifying vision of the whole ladder extension separating from the building and clattering down, much as the padlock had.

Then she reached the first platform, got to her feet, and looked down.

He was already there, at the bottom. Axe in hand, gazing up at her.

He doesn't know what to do.

Freya said nothing. She fought for breath; she wiped away tears and snot; she got her breath back; she ached from every cut and scratch, at every joint.

'I *could* come on up,' he said, out of breath himself. 'But you'd have a clear advantage. I could go and get my shotgun, but you'll be long gone by the time I get back. And, fair play to you, Freya. I set the game, and you won it. You won it. The first one to do so. There comes a time you just have to take your hat off.'

He laid the axe down at his feet. Then he straightened up and applauded, muffled reports that echoed out into the darkness as his gloves came together.

'Bravo, lass.'

Then he picked up the axe and padded away the way he had come. From higher up, Freya could see an opening in the ground, like a subway entrance, with steps leading down underground. She must have run close enough to fall down the steps; another lucky break.

That's where he had come from, and likely how he had managed to get the drop on her on top of the roof. The place must have been a warren of them, and he knew them all.

Freya stayed put. The only danger was if he *did* come back with his shotgun. But for him, that was a risk. All Freya had to do was hit the open ground and get running. The site was ring-fenced, but even in the gloom, and from a distance, she could see the gaps in it. Behind that, some forest. And if she made it to the forest, he would have to be supernaturally lucky to find her.

Freya had a sudden flashback to Cheryl Levison's bare

feet, and the pain she must have felt running on loose stones without shoes. He'd handicapped her, Freya thought. Levison had been fit and strong, and too much of a risk.

He hadn't hobbled Freya. He had underestimated her fitness. And that was his mistake.

Then nausea struck home. She sobbed, running her hair through her hands. 'I'm so sorry,' she said, gazing towards the hill where the bunker lay. 'I'm sorry. I couldn't help you. I'm sorry. I'm sorry…'

She would stay put and keep watch. Freya had no idea of the time – her watch, and of course her phone, were long gone. But he could not stay here forever. Not with a body to dispose of.

Freya heard a crackle of flame. Fingers of fire tickled the edge of the pit, surely coming from the roof of the bunker – too bright, surely using petrol or some other accelerant.

The bastard could smoke me out.

But he didn't. A moment or two later, on the other side of the pit, a pair of headlights came on. It was the white van; the lights flashed twice, as if in farewell. Then the van reversed out, and headed back along the supply route, winding its way around a hill and then disappearing out of sight.

57

She waited until it grew light, then clambered down. The smoke from the fire had brought no attention, climbing high into the still air. But surely it had been spotted from a road, somewhere. But no one came, and it burned itself out. Thankfully there was no stench, either – though possibly he had removed what remained of Cheryl Levison. Despite a life that had lately been filled with unusual experiences, Freya had never smelled burning human flesh, and it was hardly an ambition.

She dropped to the ground, every ache amplified as she loped away from the crane – away from the tiny road they had come in on, past the chasm of the quarry, and into a forested area beyond a patchy iron link fence. This, too, was dangerous. Knowing how sly and well prepared he was, if there was a secondary ambush to mop her up, then this is where he lay in wait. It was overgrown, without any obvious path through the trees. She followed her nose – or more specifically, her ears – towards a very faint sound of running water.

She came to a river, a natural twist in the ground, with lots of stepping stones in the form of slabs probably blasted from the quarry. She skipped across, and then she heard the traffic.

There was a main road nearby, but Freya emerged onto a lonely single-carriageway route, a place without crash barriers. Soaking wet, tired and hurt, she waited by the side of the road.

It took a while for any cars to come past. She signalled one, but it was a tiny car driven by a tinier woman, and Freya caught a look of sheer alarm as she speeded up, weaving into the middle of the road to get out of the way.

'I suppose I look a fright,' she muttered. Then she cried a little.

She had better luck with the next vehicle: a lorry. It had a load of live chickens, and the stench was awful as it went past; but the brake lights came on, and the truck stopped, hazards blinking, while she ran up to the cab.

It was a darling old man, surely past retirement age. His bald head creased in worry. 'You all right, there? I thought I was looking at a ghost or something, when I spotted you!'

Freya told a story about a mountain biking trip going wrong, having an accident and her bike being useless – not completely false, now that she considered it – and complained of being hurt and needing a ride home. He hadn't asked any other questions, but allowed her to drink from a flask. *Fine irony if the Woodcutter turned out to be nobody. If I should take a drink from a drugged flask, then wake up back where I started.*

But she didn't. She was soon back in the city, where the old man implored her to go to hospital and get her cuts and scrapes checked. She gave him a kiss on the forehead, and walked back home, where she was particularly struck by how little attention she drew from the masses, desperately minding their own business. Despite the tears streaming down her face, and an alarming twitch that had developed in her lower lip. The pain had come in, too, dreadful sparks going through her knee and ankle joints. At one point she stopped, and hunkered down to relieve an awful cramp. People simply flowed around her. Freya supposed she might have done the same.

She had a spare key planted behind a cracked section of brick outside. She let herself in, turned on every light, screamed aloud before she hurled open each and every cupboard, poked underneath the bed with a broom handle and was particularly vicious with every pair of curtains before she was satisfied that she was absolutely, positively alone. Then she blessed the negligence that had meant she kept her landline, called Tamm, and barely got past the first few sentences before her cries became hysterical, and the pain in every injury became unbearable.

Finally he calmed her and got the details. 'Wait – a quarry, you said? An old excavator? I know exactly where that is. Don't worry, Freya. I'm coming round.'

When he was there – just him and a kind-looking female officer who might have been younger than she was – he listened to her intently.

'Did you find her?' Freya asked.

Tamm only nodded.

'There was nothing I could do, nothing, I swear to God…'

'There's nothing anyone could do,' he said. 'There's no blame, no guilt, with someone that black-hearted. Someone so lacking. He's not even human.'

'I thought when he fell, he might have broken his neck. I thought it was over.'

'Did you see anything – eye colour, skin, anything?'

'I can't even be sure of the skin colour. Couldn't tell you his height, exactly.'

'Was there anything you recognised? Inflection, pattern of speech, anything?'

She shook her head. Then she looked less certain. 'I can't be sure.'

'What's your gut feeling? Tell me.'

'I… I can't be sure. Was it him? Was it my dad?'

Tamm swallowed. 'We don't know. We're going to speak to him now. It's highly unlikely, but we'll soon find out.'

'Whoever it is, I think I can catch him,' Freya said. 'I think there's a way. But we'll need to be quiet about it.'

58

Glenn was nervous when he appeared at the door of the pub. Freya was sat underneath the immense red and silver coffee machine, perched on top of a glass-fronted counter, her face nestled among a tempting display of pastries. When he saw her, his jaw dropped. 'God almighty… are you all right?'

'I'll live.' She smiled as he sat down.

'You didn't say anything about being hurt…' He reached out and touched her arm.

'Ah it's nothing, just cuts and scrapes when I fell over. No serious damage. Lost my bike, that's the most annoying thing. At least I managed to back up my phone.'

'Can I get you a drink? I know it's early…'

She shook her head. 'I've got things to do, today.'

'Well… Gads, why don't you move in with me?' He blurted it out with such gauche charm that she giggled. It was the first time she'd giggled in a long while.

'Bit forward, mister!'

'I mean it. When I couldn't get in touch with you that night… I was fucking frantic. I came over to your flat. I know I shouldn't have. I didn't know where you were. I thought I'd failed you, leaving you alone, after everything that happened. You were in danger.' He shook his head, trying to clear an unpleasant thought.

'Hey. It's fine. Nothing's your fault. I didn't tell you I was going to meet my dad. You remember? So you could have been with me. Had you been there, we might all have been fine.'

'Except for Levison.'

Freya said nothing. She looked at the glass case, and their faces reflected in it.

'You seen him since?' Glenn asked.

She shook her head. 'I think it's best for all concerned that I don't see him for a while. He had an alibi for that night. It's unlikely it was him.'

'Unlikely?'

'Yeah. The concierge at the flat he stayed in can't be sure if he left by the back staircase or not late at night. But given he stayed at the restaurant on his own for a while, it's really unlikely he managed to kidnap both me and Levison in good time.'

'So, am I going to get to meet him, then?'

'Definitely. We'll have to wait until things die down, though. Or until they catch the new Woodcutter.'

'Thought it was just one Woodcutter?'

'So far as anyone knows.'

He frowned. 'You know something. Or you've heard something.'

'Just a hunch,' Freya said, with a smile.

'You're up to something,' Glenn said, frowning. 'You're planning something. I'm not sure I like it.'

'You'll find out. I'll play it close to my chest, for now. But you'll know soon.'

'Why the secrecy?'

Freya took a deep breath. 'I don't want you involved, Glenn. The person who spoke to me that night... They know who you are. And I don't think they like you very much. I think you'd be as well keeping away from the inquiry. And being as safe as you can. Can you move back to your parents' for a while? He's clever, whoever he is. He might be a berserker when he's set loose, but he's all about the planning in the run-up. And one other thing: don't pick up any loose coins or notes if you see any.'

Glenn folded his arms and eyed up her jacket, boots and rucksack. 'Where are you off to?'

'A day by myself. I'm going to visit some friends.'

'Can I come?' he said, at last.

She shook her head. 'Sorry. Single ticket, this one. I'll be in touch, Glenn. Things get too interesting when we're together. I don't think I'm wrong about that.'

He looked as if he might actually cry. 'No. Not wrong.'

'It's best you go, Glenn.'

He nodded, and then he was gone. Freya took a deep breath, checked her watch, then put on her rucksack.

The waitress, who had been annoyingly nosy while this exchange was going on, cocked her head at Freya as she got up. 'He was nice, love,' she said, brazenly. 'Not giving him up, are you?'

'Nah,' she said, smiling. 'Just letting him go, to see if he comes back.'

'Doesn't always work like that,' the waitress said. 'Take it from me.'

After paying up, Freya heaved the pack onto her back, and walked to the station.

He had followed her, of course. He didn't even try to hide it particularly well, only thinking to duck into the waiting room once Freya rounded the corner.

She beckoned to him. He approached, a shy child called out by the teacher.

'I don't think you're the best listener,' she said. 'I'm not being secretive because I want to get one over on you. I'm not doing a deal or working a hustle. It's dangerous. I can't get you involved. This is life or death, now. I can't have that… I can't think about it. I don't know how I'm going to recover. I don't know…' She couldn't say anything else. Her rucksack thudded against the concrete. She covered her face.

Glenn's hands were gentle. He took one of hers in his. 'And I'm not here for a scoop. Or an angle. Or a book deal. I'm here for you. Whatever you're going to face, I'm facing it with you.'

After a long train journey into flat, green countryside, they emerged on a rural station. 'Glad you've got your walking shoes on.' Freya indicated, as she tied the hem of her waterproofs. 'This place is out in the sticks. They all were, really.'

'So what drew you to this place?' Glenn said. 'If you didn't get any more clues, that is.'

'It's close to where Florence Ceulemans vanished. Dutch fruit picker on a gap year. It's an old industrial unit, massively overgrown… Already searched by Bernie Galvin's team, when it happened. Given the previous locations, I thought it was a good fit.'

'I never focused on Florence Ceulemans – too many other variables in that one. It makes perfect sense to me. Seems like… him.'

She nodded. 'I thought so. Gut feeling. I'd like to have a look.'

'I've not been the world's most consistent person on this, but shouldn't we get a hold of the police, now? I think our cloak-and-dagger time is up. For you it is, definitely. He already tried to kill you. We're flirting with disaster.'

'We might be. It's dangerous. I told you. And I don't want you out here. How can I make it clearer to you?'

'Surely call Tamm. Run it past him.'

'I did.' Freya looked down at the table. 'He told me he thought I was reading too much into things. He said he thought I should stay away from it all.'

'I'm not surprised,' Glenn said. 'Meddling in it, after what happened to Cheryl Levison… It's a bad idea. I think we should quit, tell the police what we know, and let them handle it. If the man's out there, they can get the place surrounded and then make an arrest.'

'He said he will look out for me, whatever that means. So there's that. Unless the Woodcutter is a policeman. Him, specifically.'

'What reasons do you have for saying that?'

Freya smiled. 'You add up the coincidences, then it seems ridiculous to call them coincidences. Showing up that afternoon when I saw the carving in the woods… That's suspicious. But it's just an idea. I don't think it's him.'

'Who do you think it is?'

'I can't say.'

'Your dad?'

There was a long silence before Freya shook her head. 'Not him. I might be wrong. It's just an idea. But I think today's the day we find out.'

'You're planning something. Not just a search.' He frowned. 'Spill it.'

'I've invited one or two people out here to meet us. I think one of them, or both of them, is the Woodcutter. You'll see soon enough. I've got an idea how he operates. How he's been killing people. How he catches them. Everything. But today is the end to it. I think we can bring the Woodcutter down. And if we're clever, no one gets hurt.'

'You have to at least tell me…'

'I can't, Glenn. You'll see soon enough. I've got my reasons.'

'It's in case it's me, isn't it?' He looked angry, now. 'That's why you won't say. You can't be sure.'

Freya shook her head. She couldn't answer that. Because she didn't want to lie. *He'd know*.

She turned to the window and watched her reflection, scratched a thousand times by the blurred trees outside. *If only I could slow my heart just a little*, she thought. *Just a tiny bit*.

The station was unmanned, and deserted. After consulting her new phone, Freya took Glenn along an overgrown path, where every flicker of greenery seemed to conceal an assassin. It was an odd day for July; cool out, with cloud cover and spots of rain. It was the time of day that might have been unpleasant for being overcast, but it felt more like early October than the height of summer.

The path stretched out, taking in farmland, then forest. Soon they reached an open area where some buildings had once stood, but which were now not even rubble. Just the outlines of various structures remained on a grid pattern across an expanse of concrete, threaded with upstart weeds grown to freakish height. The landscape was flat, leading towards trees on the horizon, with only two or three small storage buildings or even outhouses clinging to the far end of the foundations.

'Online mapping's telling me nothing,' Glenn said, glancing at his phone. 'You said this was an industrial unit?'

'Yeah. What you're looking at used to be a fat-processing plant.'

'What's that?'

'Somewhere you change animal fat into useful things. Can be made into all sorts of products. Gummy sweets; creams; soaps; cooking oil; they don't waste anything. It went out of business years ago. Still smells a bit. No one's sure why. Maybe there's some underground storage facility that was left there everyone forgot about it.

'Nice.'

'I think there's been some planning permission lodged to build houses, but that's all.'

'So where's our visitors?' Glenn said. 'I feel like we're totally exposed out here.'

'No sign of them yet. But I'd probably hide, if I was them.'

'Those buildings over there look a good bet. Maybe too obvious?' Glenn set his jaw. He reached into his backpack, and pulled out a baseball bat.

Freya's eyes widened.

'Don't worry,' he said, dismissively, 'not quite the Woodcutter's weapon of choice, is it?'

'Close enough.' Freya kept her voice low. 'Maybe keep it out of sight. We have to assume we're being watched.'

'Yeah, about that. Shouldn't the cops be watching us anyway?'

'Unless Tamm's the killer.'

Glenn stopped. 'Is Tamm the killer?'

'I doubt it... I don't know.' For the first time, she didn't. Freya had expected to have company already, but there was no sign of it. The silence of the place, the dearth of any sign of human activity, was beyond strange now, and into the weird. *Someone's here, she thought. Someone's waiting, quietly. I should not have played a game. This was stupid.*

Glenn tried to stay composed, but his lip trembled as he spoke. 'If the Woodcutter ambushes us, though – what then? We don't stand a chance.'

'There's always a chance if there's two of us,' Freya said, not sounding anything like as brave or forthright as she'd intended. 'Plus – we're out in the open.'

'You said he used a shotgun, though.'

'Did I?' Freya leapt, almost at the sound of her own voice. 'I'm not sure I did.'

'You did. You told me everything.'

Freya rubbed her forehead, and shivered. 'Maybe I did. Maybe I'm losing my mind. Follow me – and stick to a clear path. He might have this place snared.'

'You serious?'

She didn't answer.

Glenn followed her towards the block graph row of

buildings close to the trees. Wisteria and bindweed in full white bloom snaked across the red brick structures. As they grew closer, they could see that one squat building had no door, but a network of pipes inside. Whatever its purpose was, it was long defunct. Aside from that, there were two other buildings, one of which looked like a standard shed with windows, and another that looked like it might have housed an electricity relay station.

Freya almost lost her nerve. Gripping the handles on her rucksack, she fought an urge to cast it to the cracked concrete and take to her heels, back up the path, back towards the creepy railway station, up the track if need be, until there were people and shelter and an absolute end to this madness.

Glenn stopped. 'There's someone there,' he said.

'Which one?' Freya narrowed her eyes.

'The shed. The brickwork one. It looks like something the three pigs built. The door's open.' He whispered, and crouched. '*Dear sweet Jesus I can see something move. Someone's in there.*'

Freya didn't join him. She stared hard at the building Glenn had described. Was there someone there? At the window? 'Let's keep going. Slowly.'

'We can't just walk up to it!' Glenn hissed.

'We can. The time for games is over. Let's see who it is.' She looked at her hand; it shook, way beyond normal. She made it into a fist, and kept going.

Taking each step as if they were traversing a creaking ice floe, they moved towards the end of a long, risen area where a building must have stood. The open doorway was visible, past a groping hand of overgrown weeds. And there, they could see a pair of booted feet, supine, toes upward, blocking the door.

'Don't like those weeds,' Glenn said, through a clenched jaw. 'Behind us. Don't like them at all. Not a great fan of those trees, either.'

'If there's someone there, they must be lying flat.'

'It's possible, though.'

'We've no choice, now.' Turning towards the shed, Freya called: 'Hello?'

'Who's there?' came a weak, muffled reply.

'Careful,' Glenn said, the bat in his hand. 'Stay back.'

Before she could protest, Glenn reached the door first, jaw tensed. Freya nodded at him. He touched the door. It creaked open fully.

The figure of a man was sat in the doorway, with an oat-coloured burlap bag over his head. The taper towards the top was almost comical, as if the man sat there had been placed in a dunce cap. He was sat with his back against the far wall of the shed in the dirt and grime of the floor, with his hands behind his back.

'Who's there?' the voice croaked.

'Who's asking?' Freya asked, glancing around.

'Is that… Freya Bain?'

She approached the figure, and cautiously removed the hood.

Underneath was Mick Harvie. His face was bruised and cut in several places. He winced against the light, and spat straw and old grass onto the ground. 'Get out of here,' he said. 'He's here. He's going to kill us all. I think he left me here as bait. Get out of here, as quick as you can, I mean now, don't wait, he's…'

'Who?' Glenn asked.

'Who do you think, genius?'

There was a rustle, yes, from the undergrowth behind them as a figure got to its feet. 'You out to chop some wood, boy?' someone leered.

Mick Harvie's head sunk. 'It's too late. I told you. He put me here as bait,' he whispered. 'None of us stands a chance now.'

Someone came into the light from the trees. He held a shotgun on them.

'No,' Freya said, raising her hands. 'That's not right. That's not it at all.'

'Nobody fucking move. Not one of you,' said Bernard Galvin.

59

Galvin's eyes looked as if they had been bored into his skull. In the bright sunshine, his skin had the texture of a tangerine; in places he looked like he had been burned.

'Great that you're all here,' he sneered. 'I would like a really calm, clear explanation, for why you brought me out here to this shithole, Freya, and presented me with this human skid mark, here.'

He kicked Harvie's feet, and the latter cringed, turning away. His hands must have been bound behind his back.

Freya licked her lips, her eyes on the shotgun. Galvin covered them all with it. 'The reason I brought you out here is because I wanted to get down to the nitty-gritty. By the time I go to bed tonight, I want to know who it is. I had thought Cheryl Levison was involved – absolutely sure of it, in fact. But she's off the list of suspects. One of the people I invited here is the Woodcutter. And I know who it is.'

'You better spit it out, then,' Galvin said. 'And when you tell me who it is, I'll spread him all over that back wall. What's this runt doing here?'

'I invited him. Same as you,' Freya said. 'You were top of the list. Mainly because of the pop gun you keep getting out. Highly inappropriate, that.' She nodded towards the shotgun, which he had angled towards the concrete foundations, the stonework appearing blond in a sudden burst of sunshine. 'Plus, you know... whenever there's a miscarriage of justice, someone benefits. You benefited, in the case of my dad. All the kudos of catching a killer. When the conviction was proven to be unsafe. That was suspicious, Bernie. You must admit. Maybe there's more than self-preservation at play.'

She could barely say it, she was so scared, her voice oscillating in and out of normal pitch. She had heard the phrase "cold sweat", but never knew the truth of it until now, across her forehead, at her armpits. Her guts began a mad dance.

'Freya...' Glenn warned.

'Plus, Bernard, it has to be said – you're a bit of a maniac. Even poor old Mick here used to stick up for you, you know. Until you gave him the black eye and stuff. His face is still a mess. God's sake, that was proper psychotic behaviour. You're not right, Bernard.'

Mick Harvie's one good eye darted in his skull. 'Freya, don't wind him up, for Christ's sake.'

'You think it was me?' Galvin snorted. 'It couldn't have been me, you silly bitch. I've got alibis all over the place. Notebooks and records that put me at work, or at my house with my family, when the killings took place. How could I be the Woodcutter? Think about it, lass.'

'There's something about you screams "headcase" to me. And I know the type, let me tell you. Why did you batter Mick again?'

'I didn't batter Mick,' Galvin said. 'When I came down here he was already tied up, with a bag over his head.

Thought the twat was dead, to tell you the truth. Till he whimpered something. Didn't you, Mick?' Galvin kicked Harvie's feet again.

Then Galvin raised the gun again, this time pointing it between Freya and Glenn. They both instinctively raised their hands.

'Bernard, if you value your life, put that gun down. I'm serious.'

'Value my life?' he cackled. 'More than you value yours? You're not making a bit of sense. Why are we out here? What is it you want to find out, and how do you plan to do it?'

'I'll tell you,' Freya said. 'First you have to lower the gun, really slowly. We're not armed. Are we, Glenn?'

'That looks like a baseball bat to me,' Galvin said, nodding at Glenn's hand. 'You looking to play some games, son?'

Glenn simply dropped the bat, and said nothing.

'OK. Good. I'm in charge, here. No ifs, no buts. Now you say you don't know what's going on. Harvie, here, told me you invited him out here, too. If this is some kind of set-up for the press, or some kind of photo opportunity, I'm warning you…'

'Nothing so dramatic,' Freya said. 'I've got a friend positioned out here. A policeman.'

'Is that a fact?' Galvin said, in mock wonderment.

'I can't be sure that he's any good with a gun, but he's probably brought along someone who's excellent with one. Better than you are with a shotgun, I bet. So for your own sake, put the gun down, Bernard.'

'Sounds like a bluff,' Galvin said.

'I set this meeting up,' Freya said. 'Think about it, Bernard. You think I came here without backup? There's a detective out there. He's been here since lunchtime. Put the gun down, and you won't get shot out of your brogues.' As Freya said this, her knees felt as if they were going to sag, in sheer stress, and the pain of hope. Please be there, Tamm. Please be there. 'I'm not joking. There's another reason for it, too.'

Galvin smiled. 'Well. What have I got to lose? I'll play.' He dropped the shotgun, and stepped away from it.

'That was sensible,' Freya said. She felt sweat drip down the back of her neck.

'So, what now?' Galvin said.

'Come over here and stand beside us.'

'What? What for?'

'Just do it, Bernie. Please. You're not safe. *Isn't it fucking obvious?*'

'Don't talk in riddles,' Galvin snapped. 'What's your plan?'

'I think the plan is for you to close your mouth, forever,' Mick Harvie said.

'What did you say, runt?' Galvin sneered, baring his teeth.

Then Mick Harvie sprang forward. His hands weren't tied; had never been tied. Galvin reacted fast, groping for the shotgun – but not fast enough.

Harvie had his own shotgun. He raised it a split second before Galvin could do the same. Harvie grinned.

For a surreal second, Harvie had the barrel jammed against Galvin's groin, the latter staring at it in complete stupefaction. Then Harvie pulled the trigger.

Galvin grunted like a sow, and took off. The angle of his hips contracted at an unnatural angle, and he fell to the ground. His off-grey anorak was spattered with blood, as was his face. Red streaks were torn across his wide-open mouth. He bucked and writhed, falling to the side, then turning onto his face, hands twitching.

Mick Harvie came in behind him, placed the barrel against Galvin's backside, and fired again.

Galvin's hips buckled. He uttered a choked scream, which soon turned to a gurgle, then grew silent. His grey eyes were open, stark and wide, as if utterly incredulous.

Freya was on the floor, tasting dust, her nose squashed painfully into concrete. Glenn was on top of her… *Shot?* No – he'd thrown himself over her. Protecting her. He rolled off, and they both looked up.

Harvie grinned at Freya. 'What was the quote, again? What did Bernie say to me? "Did you ever really want to do something for years, then just do it?" That's what the man said, wasn't it? That day, at his house?'

Harvie reversed the shotgun, then smashed the stock into the dead man's face, once, twice, three times, enormous blows, obliterating the features. Freya saw teeth, flecks of bone, and a single eye, dislodged from a socket. She whimpered, and covered her face.

'There we go!' Harvie said, after the seventh or eighth blow. He was spattered with blood. It showed on his teeth as he grinned. 'That's the end of that. What victim is he, Freya? Where are we up to now?'

'You tell us,' she whispered. She looked to the ground, all the while thinking: *Tamm. Surely to God, Tamm is here. Surely I wasn't wrong.*

'You're kidding,' Glenn said. 'This guy here – the reporter. He's the Woodcutter?'

'Yes. It's him,' she said. And then she dared to look at his blood-streaked, grinning face. *It's the first proper smile he ever gave. He looks like he means it.* Her lips were twitching, her thighs shuddering, as if she was out in the cold.

'The original and best,' Harvie said, spreading his arms, as if acclaiming the crowd. 'You could call this an exclusive interview. What was it that tipped you off, Freya, out of interest?'

'Loads of things. Mainly it was the boat,' Freya said. 'I'd seen it on your driveway. First time I met you. Someone had to use a boat to get those bodies to the weir; you had one. But your height and build tipped me off, too. Galvin was too squat. Glenn was about the same size, but broader; Tamm was too tall. He had to be someone closely connected to me, I was thinking. He was following me too closely. An ex-copper might have had those kind of spooky skills. Or an experienced, old-school hack. One with a thing for murder cases.

'Then, there was your original source, the one you tipped me off about in the first few days... Glenn had access to police files through informants, and you told me this before the first report was filed on the new Woodcutter case. I thought you might have been ahead of the curve. You knew too much. The tip-offs, the double-crosses... You had too much knowledge. Then, that night at the quarry, you mentioned me kicking you in the balls, that time you doorstepped me. On top of that, if there was anyone I'd just met who knew where I lived and was stalking me... It was most likely you. I had already caught you doing it. And the clincher – that new injury you have, on top of the bruises when Galvin smacked you one. I did that. When you tried to grab me. At the cabin.'

Harvie scratched his chin. 'I was a bit careless, with the boat. But then I've been careless all round. Bit like when I let you twat me with that brass slat, or whatever it was.' He tapped his face, beneath the purple and yellow shiner. 'Almost got me right in the eye. Could have been game over right there. You're a clever lass. Fair play. Now, that just leaves the question of who our mystery guest is. Because I'll tell you what… He isn't that policeman. Tamm, that was his name, wasn't it?'

Freya said nothing. She felt nausea in the pit of her stomach, making a fist and knocking on the door of her gullet. The sweat on her neck was now as cool as chilled raw meat. She shared a glance with Glenn; he looked like he was actually crying, his raised hands quaking out of control.

Harvie held the shotgun on them – *how many shots? If only two, he's used them…* She didn't like the grin. She'd never liked it. Now it had an extra edge, a leer. 'You see – Tamm wasn't hiding out there.' He reached into the dusty doorway. 'He's hiding in here. I set up shop here almost as soon as you called me. He got here at first light. Worse luck.'

Harvie hurled something from the doorway. The curve – the arc of descent – was narrow. The object spun, the long hair like a dervish.

It landed two feet from them.

The too-long hair obscured the face, mercifully, except for the distended, open jaw – a mockery of animation. But there was no doubt that this was Tamm's head.

Freya had no idea when she started screaming. She might have been about to faint; she was aware of a strong presence behind her. Glenn; Glenn with tears in his eyes; Glenn terrified; but Glenn, practically holding her up.

'Hold on,' he whispered. 'Think it through. We'll get our chance.'

'Ah, knock it off,' Harvie sneered. 'God, you get sick of the screaming in this game, that's the only drawback. I guess some people like it, I don't know… Anyway. I'd like to get started here. Unless there are some more special guest stars to come?'

'You might be lucky.' Freya forced the words from a throat that felt glued shut. 'You just might.'

60

Still holding the shotgun on them, Harvie reached into one of the bushes hemming in the raw-guts brickwork of the shed. 'I'm going to kill you,' he said, conversationally. 'But I'll get some answers first. I just don't know who I'm going to torture first, to make the other one talk. Usually I'd go with "ladies first", to make the man crack, but you look about as wet as they come, son.'

Glenn's face was out of control, his eyes glassy with tears. Maybe a step or two away from hitting his knees and begging. 'Run,' he said to Freya, out of the corner of his mouth. 'We have to take our chances and run. I'll make sure if he shoots, he shoots me.'

'No,' Freya said.

'Go on, then,' Harvie said, raising the shotgun. 'Run.'

Freya raised her hands, and stepped in front of Glenn. 'I'll tell you what you need to know. Don't hurt Glenn. He doesn't know anything about it. I brought him here, same as I brought you. I knew he would try to follow me. And he did.'

'What?' Glenn gasped.

'Boy's right to be curious,' Harvie muttered. 'Why did you bring him?'

'Help. If I needed it.'

Harvie tilted his head at an odd angle as Freya approached. 'Something fishy about you, lass. Too much of your father in you by halves.'

'You may be right about that. But, you first. Tell me about the Woodcutter.'

'I'm the fucking Woodcutter,' he snarled.

'Yeah, I mean the *other* Woodcutter. Come on, Mick. You were practically falling over yourself to tell us about it. What was the message you left at the weir? "To Me, To You?" It's obvious, now. *There were two of you*. There must have been. Let someone loose, and take the chance of chasing them on your own? There are a million ways that could have gone wrong. And it's not like we're in Alaska, or the Amazon, or somewhere like that. Even in the far north of Scotland, you've got a decent chance of bumping into people out on the mountains. That's how you did it, didn't you? One chases, the other one waits at the target zone you gave them. Isn't that right?'

'I was the architect,' Harvie said, proudly. 'I planned it all out. We both executed it – I'll give you that.'

'Except for the squaddie. What was the story there?'

'Ah! Now, that was the hardest one. The odd one out. I took him on myself. One-man job. Took a swing at me outside a court martial case I was covering. Nasty little fucker. He paid the price, though. You can be as fast or as hard as you like – I corner you with a shotgun, you've fucking had it. He was still alive when I chopped him, though. I enjoyed that. More than I enjoyed braining everyone's favourite corrupt policeman, over there. Your dad should be thanking me for that one.'

'Who was it?' Glenn said, perhaps reassured on some level by the friendly tone of the conversation. 'If there were two of you, who was the other Woodcutter?'

'Gads, he's really keen on this case, isn't he? In the face of grim death, he has to know. Not as bright as he makes out, though.' Harvie cackled. 'Patience, lad. I'll tell you before you die. OK? That's a promise.'

'If there're two Woodcutters, the other one was Galvin, surely,' Glenn said. 'He was top of my list. He tied everything together.'

'That bastard?' Even though his nemesis lay dead and still bleeding just yards away, Harvie couldn't conceal his venom. 'It would have been a good ruse, all the same. Him belting me one. If we'd made it look like we were enemies, but actually we were in it together. I can see your thinking. Best acting I've ever done, that afternoon. Talk about biting your lip and taking it. You will never know the fury I had to bottle in. Well... Maybe you've just seen the fury, actually. But no. It wasn't Bernie. He was a psychopath, though. The worst kind, in my book, and I've got the fucking expertise when it comes to that – one who thinks he's doing the right thing. Me – I'm a scumbag. I just enjoy hunting and killing people. Always have. My mother was terrible to me, as well. I wet the bed and I got bullied at school. I've read all the books, too. Big deal. Boo hoo, blah fucking blah.

'Bottom line, however I got here – I like it. This is leisure. This is what I do for a hobby. But guys like Galvin... When they get in charge of things, that's when it becomes systemic. When some coppers fit you up, they say it's something to do with confirmation bias, or selection bias. They've just gone with the information that fits their theories, and ignored the evidence. That idiot just wanted someone in jail, and to look good in the papers. In so far as someone so butt-ugly can look good. He's prettier now, in fact. Anyway. Take a good look where that level of scheming gets you. I struck a blow for justice, and that's the truth. Several blows, in fact.'

Glenn had backed away, just an inch or two, while Harvie was focused on her. Freya tried not to make eye contact with him. They still had a weapon. Had Harvie forgotten?

'So, you give me something now. Who's your candidate for my little helper?'

'You killed her,' Freya said. 'Cheryl Levison.' Her voice crumpled upon saying that name. She remembered the axe splitting the bedframe up above her in that filthy rathole of a bunker. She remembered the gurgling sound as Levison's last breaths escaped. She remembered contorting into a ball, too terrified to move. She remembered the blood, a rain of it, dripping onto the floor. The smell of it. She sobbed.

'I chopped Cheryl Levison up, all right,' Harvie said, chuckling. 'But you're off beam. She wasn't involved. I just had to get rid of her. Your dad, you see… Your dad might have let something slip to her. Every chance of it. Good-looking woman like that, she knows how to manipulate a man. She had to go. She was my top target, but I'd have taken you, just as easily. Nice surprise for your dad, on the day of his release! Too bad I couldn't have sorted you both. And, think about it – Levison's a little too young to be involved in the originals. And she wasn't involved in the new cases. All my own work, those ones. You wouldn't believe how much I got into those… Well, you would believe it, in fact. You were there!'

'Right up until you killed her, I thought Levison was there to help you, that night.'

Harvie threw his head back and laughed. 'What a load of old bollocks! That doesn't make a bit of sense. God, it's so obvious who the other Woodcutter was. I get the feeling you just don't want to admit it.'

The shotgun dropped, just a little. *This might be the time.*

'Yeah. It is obvious. And always was.'

Harvie showed his teeth, a cartoonish grin. 'That's my girl. Say it, go on. Out loud. Do it for me.'

She shook her head. 'You have to explain it first. My dad went to jail. He could have put you in there with him. Why didn't he?'

'Vanity.' Harvie grinned. 'In a nutshell. Guy's a rock star, and he knows it. Handsome, oversexed little shit, back then. One thing I never got to the bottom of – guy as good-looking as that, why does he feel the need to chop women up? You should have seen them outside court. Think the Beatles landing in America for the first time. It was fucking embarrassing, the way those bitches lost their minds. Grown goddamned women in Laura Ashley floral print fucking dresses. Placards. "I Believe Him". Good Christ in his kingdom.'

'That doesn't answer why he didn't just blame you. He went inside.'

'Loyalty, in a nutshell. Or something like it.' He shook his head. 'Oh, come on. You're still defending him? He's the other Woodcutter. Your dad. All along. We were partners!'

'Nonsense,' Freya croaked. 'Why in God's name would he go to jail... to protect you?'

'It's complicated. The thing is, your instincts were kinda

right. You dad's a maniac, no quibbles there. But he's got some good in him. You see, your dad had this guilt, shame, remorse, call it what you like. Maybe "the thing I lack" is the best description. I couldn't give a shit. I'm a sicko. I got back into it in later life, as a solo act! Ha! But he hated himself. For indulging his urges. Common thing. You don't have to be a Catholic to be guilty here, but it helped in his case. He didn't want to carry on with it. So he decided to go inside, to take himself away from the urge. Justice had nothing to do with it. He took his porridge. And he didn't want to give me away. Vanity played its part. Also loyalty. We made a pact. We were friends.

'It suited me, 'course it did. But it suited him, too. It was his idea. He didn't care about the morality, as such, of what I was doing. He just wanted to be locked up for it, kept away from society. I mean my God, if you'd seen his face after he chopped those women up, I mean… the *glee*. Ever wanted to chop someone up? Imagine if it was your thing, your big goal in life. Imagine achieving it four times. He was good with the axe, as well. Credit to him for that. One chop, wallop, there's an arm. There's a thigh, cut right through. There's some fucker's head. And there's their head again, but this time, halved down the middle. He was a genius with it. An artist at work. Well.' Harvie sighed. 'In other circumstances I'd suggest going for a pint, now. I'm parched after all that talking. Best we get started.'

'Wait,' Glenn said, 'wait a minute. It was Gareth Solomon all along? I thought you said it was Levison.'

'I didn't think it was Levison, really,' Freya said to him. Her neck and shoulders were tense, and she spoke through clenched teeth. 'I was buying some time.'

Harvie's grin faded.

'You'll soon see, Glenn,' Freya said. She pointed right at Harvie, then, gazing into his eyes, her teeth gritted. '*You* won't, though.'

Harvie looked uncertain, for a second. He paused, turning his head slightly.

Just as the axe crashed into it.

His legs buckled, and he fell on his backside. He blinked; there was no blood yet, but the axe was buried in the side of his face, splitting the cheekbone and some of the temple. Its handle was parallel to the vertical line of his body.

Harvie tugged at it uselessly, then sank forward, his backside resting against the brickwork of the shed.

He gurgled, and it is possible that the last thing he saw was Gareth Solomon, snatching up the shotgun from his lap and hurling it away.

Then Solomon grabbed the axe handle, placed a boot against Harvie's ruined face, and tugged the axe free with a clean snap.

Harvie's head lolled back, resting against the brickwork, jaw dropped wide, as the blood surged down the side of his face. Harvie might have been dead by then; he certainly was after Solomon centred himself, legs braced, and swung hard at his face.

The horizontal axe blade swept clean through his mouth, shearing through the cheeks, embedding itself in the back of the mouth and clean through the other side. The blade buried itself into the brickwork with a clean, metallic chime and a puff of dust.

Harvie, the axe handle jutting from the red ruin of his cheeks at a perfect right angle, was transfixed to the wall, eyes staring, but sightless. The jaw, completely unhinged, drooped obscenely.

Solomon sighed, placing a hand on the arch of his back. 'I'm well out of practice, so sorry. I mean, I work out, but I'm old, now. And there's no substitute for active duty in the field, I find.'

Freya couldn't speak for a second or two. All she could say was, 'Hey, Dad.' She stood, tensed, fists clenched, unsure what to do. Then she pounded her own temples. Stupid. Stupid. Stupid. She knew it was a possibility, all along. But she'd believed him. Believed all the lies, thought she saw a spark of light in his eyes, wanted to believe he was innocent, ignored the obvious, the blatant facts, even as she'd recited them to him in prison. He was the killer. Maybe the worst of the two.

The glee. Those had been Harvie's words. *The glee* of it.

The horror she'd felt upon seeing the name of her father in those old newspaper reports and badly scanned photocopies… his face, chin tilted down, caught perfectly in a saturnine expression by a tabloid photographer… The thought of sharing her genes with a killer, a maniac. It was all true.

'Stop that, now,' Solomon said, blankly. 'Don't be doing that to yourself. You – four eyes – yeah, you, haircut, whatever. Put an arm round her or… whatever you do.'

Glenn did as he was told. Freya sagged into him, sobbing.

Solomon considered Harvie for a second, biting one side of his mouth and then the other. He might have been considering a frozen-over windscreen, and working out how to chisel off the ice. 'For the record… I'm sorry about

Mick,' he said. 'It's true, what he said. All of it. We had a bond. Birds of a feather. But I guess he had to go. He's left some mess. I could not *believe* he had started killing again. He must have kept that bottled up for twenty-five years. My God, can you imagine that? Unless he got really good at stalking and killing. Anyway. Now he's a great big mess, isn't he? I'm not sure how we take care of him. Or this.' Solomon tapped the edge of the axe handle with the tip of his index finger.

'You can't get away with this,' Glenn said. 'See sense.'

Solomon glared at Glenn; the younger man actually flinched.

'You didn't tell me... you had a *boyfriend*!' Solomon roared, his voice echoing out. 'Who's this drip? The famous fucking Glenn Allander from sickos dot com?'

'He's a friend,' Freya said, quickly. 'He's fine. He won't say anything.' Now she felt terror again – somehow, a worse terror than she'd felt with Harvie, or with Galvin pointing a shotgun at them. Solomon seemed more out of control. That person who'd been contained behind the reinforced glass was now on the loose. And there was no telling what'd happen to them, now. Even his own daughter. Maybe it wouldn't matter who it was, when his blood was up. She had a nauseating realisation of how he would look in the moonlight; the broad, pale face, and the staring eyes, darker than shadow.

'I'll decide who says what, my girl.' He kept his eyes on Glenn for a long time, before prodding Bernie Galvin's body with his boot. 'I am not sorry about this sack of shit, all the same. I didn't get to thank Mick for that. That's his parting gift. We'll raise a glass to him later, eh?'

'How'd you slip your markers with the police?' Freya said.

'They aren't actually watching me. If they are, well...' He spread his hands. 'It's over today, one way or the other. Mick was right about that other thing, the guilt and what have you. As well as the vanity. I'm old enough to accept all that. If we get arrested here, I'll take the credit, and I'll do the time. I was, after all, the Woodcutter. Hey – is it Glenn? Aren't you going to say hello? You have to impress your girlfriend's dad, you know. This is a very elemental moment, son. You look a little knock-kneed to be dating my daughter.'

Glenn said nothing. He stared from Freya, then back to Solomon.

'What amazes me is that the copper over there—' here he gestured towards the bloodied anemone lying in the dust a few yards away '—actually was on his own. They'd have swarmed the place by now. Just as well I arrived late, while Harvie was busy with him. Had I arrived earlier... he might have got the drop on me, the little shit. But I have to say, that was a nice bit of work. Tip of the hat to Harvie, there, so to speak. I mean we were competitive, but that doesn't mean you can't appreciate good work. Did you bring us all here, Freya?'

'I did,' she said. 'It was the best way to find out who's who. I had an idea. I just wanted to check it out.'

'You're saying you knew it was me?'

'I was in denial. Right up to the last moment. But I guess I knew, somehow. It might be an instinct. The same instinct that makes me want to speak to you, and get to know you. Maybe we're both messed up. There's a fifty-fifty chance of it, if it comes to the genes, after all.'

'Ach. That's quite sad, in a way. Very sad. We had something, maybe. That's a shame.' Solomon stared at his hands. 'Because I think… on balance… I'm going to have to kill you,' he said, almost conversationally. 'Don't get me wrong, the odds of being a free man by sunset today are non-existent. But I think… Yep, you're going to have to go.'

Glenn was braced to take off. 'Run, Freya. You first. Go.'

She shook her head. She could not make the sound with her voice, so she mouthed: *No*.

'I totally accept, I might not catch both of you. And there's a limited chance I'll get one of you, but… Yep, you've both got to go. Sorry, Freya. For what it's worth, I hope I catch him, and you get away.'

Freya locked eyes with Glenn's. 'There's another reason I picked this spot,' she said. 'I picked it because it was good and lonely.'

Solomon and Glenn both had the same expression. 'You what?'

Freya reached into her backpack, and withdrew a hatchet. The blade was polished steel, and very sharp.

Glenn's eyes appeared to be escaping from his skull. He backed off, hastily.

'I wanted someone bumped off.' Freya jerked her head towards Glenn. 'Fancy doing it for me, Daddy?'

'Are you serious?' Glenn squeaked.

'Yeah. You're too pathetic for words, Glenn. God's sake, I can't believe we did it. Daddy, I don't like my boyfriend. We can say Harvie did it.' Her eyes shone, and she grinned at him. 'Take care of it, would you?'

'Would I?' Solomon barked laughter, and rubbed his hands. 'Too bloody right! You know, you've done a perfect job with the kill site, I have to say. It's better than some of the places we staked out, back in the day.'

'Get him, Daddy.' Freya's eyes were all pupils, it seemed – black and impenetrable. They seemed to engulf the whites. She bit her lip, mock coquettishly. 'Glenn – I'd get motoring, if I was you.'

Glenn asked no questions; raised no objections. He simply started to run.

'Off he goes,' she said, absently. 'I'd like to do it, Dad. It feels right. It feels like succession.'

A grin spread across his face. He might have been crying. 'My girl,' he said.

She ran to him. He kissed her fiercely, then hugged her close.

'We going to chop him up, Daddy? Together?'

'We are.' They linked hands.

'He can't run,' Freya said, pointing towards the stumbling figure. 'I bet you could get him. Or maybe I'll get him first?'

'Killer instinct! Ha! That is a gold star for you!' He turned, and yanked the axe from Mick Harvie's still-startled death mask. Harvie finally fell forward. Though it made no odds to a corpse, the sound of his nose colliding with the concrete in the dust between his feet was wince-inducing. A red stain was turning dark on the crumbled brick at his back, and already drawing flies.

'You first,' Freya said.

'Of course, pet.'

Solomon took off. He was a sprinter; his bulk was mainly muscle, and his enormous thighs and gorilla's backside propelled him beyond Freya. The axe shone in the sunshine, sticky with gore like a butcher's parcel.

His burst of pace didn't last, and Freya soon caught up.

He was giggling in between breaths. 'I'm going to do it, do it again!' he wheezed. 'Here it comes, boy!'

Glenn ran for his life. He pleaded, he burbled, snot and tears slicked his face, and he spoke of love, even as they bore down on him. He flung up an arm; Solomon grinned.

'That's not going to help you, son! Hey, welcome to the family!'

He raised the axe over his head with both hands.

Glenn screamed.

Solomon grunted, staggered, and fell.

His axe tumbled in the dust, raising a cloud.

The hatchet Freya had swung at his leg protruded just above his right knee.

All the blood had drained from Solomon's face. Saliva trailed from his mouth. His hand closed around the hatchet, and then he screamed.

Glenn got to his feet. 'What the fuck is going on?' he said. 'I thought you were with him!'

'Of course I wasn't! I had to think fast. It was a gamble. I'm so sorry.' Freya picked up the axe. Her legs weren't working properly; she might have been walking on spokes. 'It was this or we would have had to fight him. I'm sorry. I'm sorry!' She took his face in her free hand, instinctively; he collapsed against her a moment.

'That was…' Solomon wheezed, getting onto his haunch, right leg trailing, 'well played.' He grunted, and winced. Blood wormed its way out from between the fingers of the hand clamped to the wound in thick skeins.

'Dad. Get your hand off the hatchet handle. Leave it where it is. The police will be here soon. Glenn?' She reached into her jacket, and tossed him her phone. Then she wrapped both hands around Solomon's axe handle, dragging the head back a little. Even that slight movement cut a thin furrow in the dust and concrete. It made a clean, dangerous rasp.

'You're not calling the police. Come on.' Solomon spat. Then he retched. Blood had saturated his jeans and his shoes, gathering in the dust in dark red globules like spilled wax. 'I knew it was ending today one way or the other – but come on. Not the cops.'

'Take your hand off the hatchet.' She raised the axe above her head, shoulders heaving, breathing heavily. So, so heavy. But she knew that solid mass would transmute into brute force when it fell, singing.

'I can't go back, love,' Solomon cried out as he yanked out the hatchet, and scuttled forward.

'I said, *don't*!'

Freya screamed this last word, at the top of her voice. Then she brought the axe down, hard.

61

They kept Freya waiting a long time out in the corridor. In truth it had only been a matter of weeks since she'd first arrived at this place, but it felt like ancient history. Back then, she'd only been armed with fresh knowledge; a name to go with the blank spot in her own records. Now she was armed with the truth.

To know the truth about her father left her with no guilt or shame. She was hardly the first person to have been successfully gaslit by Gareth Solomon, and probably wouldn't be the last. But the world knew, now, what he had done alongside Mick Harvie. And thanks to a leak on the police force, the world also knew that the Woodcutter's daughter had wielded the axe herself.

That was the only part she wouldn't, or couldn't face. The joy of releasing that pent-up tension, the sharp, inexorable arc, the shock of impact as the blow landed. And then Glenn's face, the utter shock, and then the revulsion, in the immediate aftermath, the phone dangling loosely from his hand.

She had not hesitated.

Was it in her? That was the question Freya might spend the rest of her life trying to answer. Was there something lurking in the genes, something affecting the mind, that she would have to live in fear of? Or even worse, was it something recessive in her, but perhaps dominant in a child she would have? Perhaps a child of hers would be pale, with dark, dark eyes. How would it feel to look into those eyes again, knowing who they belonged to? How had her mother felt?

Freya was meant to see a psychologist shortly, but she had her own armour, shield and sword by now. Her name was not Solomon; it was Bain. If need be, she could change the name again, and be something new. If Gareth Solomon's murderous instinct was precisely that – something innate, rather than inveterate – she was positive she did not have it. What she did have was her mother's compassion and fortitude. The former was the reason why she had disobeyed every instinct, and agreed to come here today.

Another non-named governor said: 'We're ready for you, Freya. You know the drill, I think.'

He was waiting for her inside another secure room, with more gorillas on the shoulders. This time, Solomon had two men stationed either side of him.

'Well. Here we are.' Freya's father sighed, and sat back.

'Yep.' Freya nodded. Despite the glass, despite the guards, she felt more insecure than she ever had in his presence. 'Right back where we started.'

'Thanks for coming. I know it can't be easy.'

'You look thinner.'

'Very nice of you to say so. I think. Weight loss is one thing to thank stress for. I never liked all the attention, really.'

Freya frowned. 'You absolutely sure about that?'

'Yeah. It's complex. I liked being the Woodcutter. But I didn't like everyone *knowing* I was the Woodcutter.'

'I think I know what you mean.' She pointed. 'I have to ask... how is it?'

Solomon raised a club-like lump of bandages, wire supports and other material coalesced around his hand in a comical hammer-like shape. 'It's a good look, I have to say. Great fun getting it through a sleeve, let me tell you. And as for wiping your bum, well... But to be honest, the leg's worse. Some amount of physiotherapy and operations for that. You're a dab hand with an axe. Dab hand... Is not a good phrase to use.'

'It's good they managed to get the hand reattached.'

'I still can't feel it. It might be the drugs. Did you really have to chop my hand off?'

'Yes.' She dropped her gaze to her hands, which had begun to wrestle one another, unconsciously. 'It should have been your neck. I had to do it. I couldn't have you hurting Glenn. Or anyone else.'

'Oh, your *boyfriend*?' He still had that edge in his voice. Freya wondered if it had ever been for comic effect, after all. 'He'd better be worth it, lass.'

'So far, so good.'

Solomon scratched his chin. 'He was going to take the heat for you. I remember that. He wanted you to get away.'

Freya found the topic genuinely uncomfortable, and dismissed it. 'He's fine. Needs a bit of work. But so does everybody. Anyway – sorry about the hand.'

'I'd say no offence, but it'd be a bit of a lie, because I'm a little bit offended that my little girl cut off my hand.'

'We were never going to have a conventional father-daughter relationship, were we?'

'I'm proud of you.' He grew serious. When he fixed Freya with that glare, she had once felt intimidated. Now, with the flesh in retreat from around his face, chin, jaw and neck, there was something haunting about it. Tragic, rather than scary. 'I mean it. You've got the right stuff. You did the right thing. But there's one thing I need you to know.'

'I'm crying again. Sorry. I didn't mean to. I said I wouldn't.'

'What I want you to know is… I wouldn't ever have hurt you. I'm not sure if you know that. I was speaking in anger, I'd never have… I mean, look how I reacted when I thought you were on my team!'

'I'm never going to know if you're telling the truth. And you're never going to get the chance to prove it. I suggest we leave it there.'

'True enough. Unless I escape.'

The guards on either side of Solomon both shuffled their feet.

Solomon grinned. 'I'm sure I won't, though. Anyway. For what it's worth, I am sorry. I lied through my teeth to you, all the way through. I wouldn't blame you for ignoring me. But if you believe only one thing that comes out of my mouth, believe that. A man like me doesn't get much in the way of blessings. But I got one in you. That's a fact.'

'Thank you,' she said.

'On top of that, you'll be happy to hear – I came clean about the other bodies.'

'Florence Ceulemans? She was the one people thought might have been killed by the Wood… by you.'

'Dutch girl. Yes.' He closed his eyes. 'Beautiful girl. I'm so sorry. Yes. Her, and four other girls. If Harvie took some on his own account, before we met, or while I was in jail, he might have taken that to his grave. I've told them everything. Tell the world, now, if you like. Tell them what I did.'

'But why?' she blurted out. 'Why did you do it? Was it just a compulsion? Did Mick Harvie manipulate you? Or did you manipulate him? How did it start? When did you know you needed to do it?'

Solomon bowed his head. 'I'm getting into it with a professional. One day I might get into it with you. Springing the lock on my mind. I can tell you it's as bad as you could imagine, and worse... And it's also an internal world you never want to know. Someday we can talk about it. Not today.'

There was silence for a second or two. Solomon broke it: 'Now. Tell me your news. What's happening?'

'I'm going to retrain. I think I'll study, take my A levels at college, then go for law school.'

'The law! Ha. Let me guess – the Levison effect?'

'Hmm, maybe not. The anti-Levison effect. I'll be a goody two shoes. That's me. Good enough to chop my dad's hand off when I thought he was doing something wrong.'

'Look forward to it. Hey, maybe I'll go to your graduation?'

'Maybe. Anyway. I was going to come here to say goodbye. But it isn't goodbye. Because I will come back. It won't be often. But I will come in and see you and speak to you. I felt a little sting, when I imagined cutting off all contact.'

'Pardon the pun.'

She grew angry. 'Just listen. Park the stupid jokes for a

minute or two. I imagined ignoring you completely. But that little pain I felt… Didn't come from you. Or me, really. It came from Mum. She would have told me that just cutting you dead was the worst thing to do. It doesn't feel right, the same way as not making contact with you in the first place felt wrong. She would have wanted me to meet you, to check in on you. If you want to talk, I'll listen. That makes me feel better. It won't be father and daughter. We'll never have chips on the beach.' Here she broke down, and her guard placed his hand on her shoulder. 'We won't have Christmases together,' she said, at last, wiping away the tears. 'But I can come here, every now and again. I don't owe you a thing. But I'll do it. Because it's right.'

Solomon seemed in shock. Did his eyes glisten, or was it just the play of harsh lighting on his oily black corneas? He sat forward, and nodded. 'That'll be just fine by me.'

He touched his forefinger to the glass. Freya instinctively pressed her own forefinger on the same spot. Then she fled.

Glenn waited at a café nearby. He ordered her an Americano, and pulled out a stool for her.

'That's that,' Freya said. 'Back to square one, I guess.'

'Was he angry with you? You know, for…' He actually mimicked a chopping motion. She burst out laughing, a positive release of tension at long last.

'Hard to say what he thought. The guy's an enigma. One day I'll get to the bottom of it all. Why he did what he did… what drives him… What he feels. If he feels anything at all. I'll keep going back. I'll talk to him. It won't be normal. It's just necessary.'

'You sure about that? God. Might be worth cutting the guy out, end of story.'

'Not a chance. He's my dad. He's my only family. It's not a case for shame. It's nothing I did. I accept it. I accept *him*. Everything he did. Everything he says. Everything he believes. I've still got a tie. I don't feel blessed. But he's all I've got. I'll never let him go.'

Glenn raised his eyebrows. 'I'm not sure I'd feel the same.'

'You don't want access, then? You don't fancy writing a bestseller?'

Glenn shook his head. 'Not if you don't want to, no. I'll go with what you want. Whatever you want, that's the right thing.'

He took her hand. She gripped it, hard.

'Glenn... genetically, I am half-maniac. And I know you're still a little bit sore about the whole chop-him-up fake-out...'

He sighed. 'We've been through that. Sore point, but, you know, I'm dealing with it...'

'But you were brave. You could have run at any point, that day. Any point at all.'

He looked towards their hands, linked on the table. 'I'd never have left you. Never.'

'Right answer. OK. Let's go for the train. And I've got an idea for tonight. Something exciting.'

He got that hopeful, puppy-dog look. 'Get into our jammies, open a bottle of wine and some crisps, and watch a really horrible documentary?'

'Perfect.' And she kissed him.

Acknowledgements

To steal from a poet, "only your undertaker knows for sure". In my case, "only your editor knows for sure", so a great big tip of the hat to Holly for her extraordinary work. This novel was a very different and difficult-to-manage creature at one stage, but she soon had it well trained. I'm very grateful for her guidance and patience.

Another tip of the hat to Helena, the peregrine falcon of copy editors. She misses *nothing*, truly extraordinary stuff. In the off chance there is an error in here, it's something I've put back in.

And a wee dram raised to Hannah – she's moved on to a new challenge in publishing, but she took a chance on me a couple of years ago at the start of this adventure. I'd been trying for years, knocking on the doors, nothing happening... Starting to wonder if it was ever going to happen... And she gave me a chance. I will never forget it. *Slainthe!*

And thanks, as ever, to Claire, Helena, Rory and Elaine, for everything.

About the Author

P.R. BLACK lives in Yorkshire, although he was born and brought up in Glasgow. When he's not driving his wife and two children to distraction with all the typing, he enjoys hillwalking, fresh air and the natural world, and can often be found asking the way to the nearest pub in the Lake District.

His short stories have been published in several books including the Daily Telegraph's Ghost Stories and the Northern Crime One anthology. He took the runner-up spot in the 2014 Bloody Scotland crime-writing competition with "Ghostie Men". His work has been performed on stage in London by Liars' League.

@PatBlack9